MW01156000

EPIDEMICS AND THE AMERICAN MILITARY

EPIDEMICS AND THE

AMERICAN MILITARY

Five Times Disease Changed the Course of War

JACK E. McCALLUM

Naval Institute Press
Annapolis, Maryland

Naval Institute Press
291 Wood Road
Annapolis, MD 21402

© 2023 by the U.S. Naval Institute
All rights reserved. No part of this book may be reproduced or utilized in any form or by any means, electronic or mechanical, including photocopying and recording, or by any information storage and retrieval system, without permission in writing from the publisher.

Library of Congress Cataloging-in-Publication Data

Names: McCallum, Jack E., author.
Title: Epidemics and the American military : five times disease changed the course of war / Jack E. McCallum.
Other titles: Five times disease changed the course of war
Description: Annapolis, Maryland : Naval Institute Press, [2023] | Includes bibliographical references and index.
Identifiers: LCCN 2023007791 (print) | LCCN 2023007792 (ebook) | ISBN 9781682477304 (hardcover) | ISBN 9781682478103 (ebook)
Subjects: LCSH: Medicine, Military —United States —History. | War —Medical aspects —History. | Communicable diseases —Transmission —History. | Epidemics —United States —History. | Smallpox —United States —Prevention —History —18th century. | Typhoid fever —Virginia —Richmond —History —19th century. | Yellow fever —Cuba —Prevention —History —20th century. | Influenza —Germany —History —20th century. | Malaria —Pacific Area —Prevention —History —20th century. | BISAC: MEDICAL / Infectious Diseases | HISTORY / Military / United States
Classification: LCC UH223 .M28 2023 (print) | LCC UH223 (ebook) | DDC 355.3/450973 —dc23/eng/20230321
LC record available at https://lccn.loc.gov/2023007791
LC ebook record available at https://lccn.loc.gov/2023007792

♾ Print editions meet the requirements of ANSI/NISO z39.48–1992 (Permanence of Paper).
Printed in the United States of America.

31 30 29 28 27 26 25 24 23   9 8 7 6 5 4 3 2 1
First printing

All maps created by Chris Robinson.

To Dana, without whose support and patience this would have been impossible

CONTENTS

ILLUSTRATIONS

ACKNOWLEDGMENTS

My gratitude to the many historians and physicians who have provided advice and the benefit of their knowledge and especially to Spencer Tucker, who started my journey with military history. I am also grateful to the editors at the Naval Institute Press, who were invaluable in making this book more accessible. Of course, any errors are mine alone.

INTRODUCTION

Four Ways to Fight an Epidemic

Humanity has but three great enemies: fever, famine, and war;
of these by far the greatest, by far the most terrible, is fever.

—William Osler, "The Study of Fevers in the South"

I n March 2020, COVID-19 broke out on the USS *Theodore Roosevelt*. The *Nimitz*-class nuclear-powered aircraft carrier was forced to return to Guam where all but a skeleton crew were removed from the ship. Ultimately 1,156 of the 4,800-man crew tested positive for the virus, and the ship's commanding officer and an assistant secretary of the Navy lost their jobs. By December, 65 percent of the Navy's deployable ships had reported cases, and although the illnesses were generally mild, operations across the fleet were curtailed by the pandemic. Some of the most sophisticated machines in history had been put out of commission by one of the simplest life forms on earth, and the only available response was quarantine—the oldest and least effective way to deal with an epidemic.

Battles are the lifeblood of military historians, and wartime epidemics have often been overlooked even though they are far from rare. The Philistine capture of the Ark of the Covenant was said to have been followed by epidemics that killed 50,000 people in 1143 BCE. A plague, possibly brought from Africa, devastated Athens in 430 BCE and led to its loss to Sparta in the Peloponnesian War. The Antonine Plague from 164–89 CE

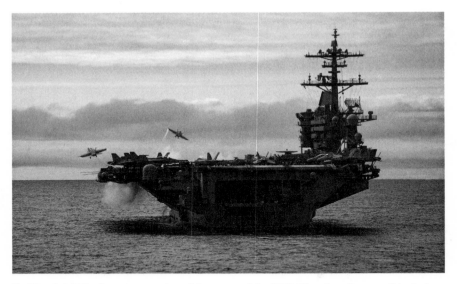

In March 2020, almost a quarter of the crew of the USS *Theodore Roosevelt* tested positive for COVID-19 and the ship was forced to return to Guam, where the crew was quarantined. *U.S. Navy*

cost Emperor Marcus Aurelius his life and marked a turning point in the wars with Germanic invaders. European crusaders managed to conquer Jerusalem in 1099, but only after losing 280,000 of their 300,000-man army, almost all to disease. Subsequent crusades fared no better, and each army brought epidemics home with them. Sequential waves of smallpox, influenza, and measles helped a small army of Spanish invaders conquer sophisticated empires in Central and South America. The Thirty Years' War saw one epidemic after another. Typhus devasted both sides from 1618 to 1630 only to be followed by bubonic plague from 1630 to 1648. Napoleon Bonaparte's armies were devastated by the Russian winter, but they suffered at least as much from Russian lice and typhus. In the Crimean War (1854–56) ten times as many British soldiers died from shigella as from Russian weapons. Twice as many Union soldiers died from disease as from wounds during the American Civil War.

That is only a sampling. It is almost impossible to find a war before the second half of the twentieth century in which contagion did not play a major part. Wars and epidemics are made for one another, and an attempt to catalog every wartime epidemic would take volumes. There are very few wars save for very brief ones in which disease has not played a role, and that role has often been decisive.

Studies of epidemic diseases also weigh down library shelves. We can neither deal with every war in which there has been an epidemic nor every disease that has complicated a war, but conflict inevitably amplifies the effects of contagion and provides unique insights into the spread and management of epidemics. We will look at selected examples.

Just as wars offer a unique perspective on epidemics, epidemics have changed wars. Infectious diseases have influenced wars' outcomes in ways that have not always been given the credit they deserve. In addition, the stunning successes against infectious disease in the last decades of the nineteenth century and the first half of the twentieth gave us an overly optimistic assessment of our ability to defeat the microorganisms that attack us. It has been almost one hundred years since the world confronted a pandemic on the scale of COVID-19, and the current pandemic has challenged that complacency. COVID-19 has reminded us that all our weapons against pandemics fall into just four categories—quarantine, ecology, pharmacology, and immunology—and none are guaranteed to be available or guaranteed to work if they are. We have been fortunate that most of the current epidemic has played out in time of peace; history has repeatedly proven that contagion is far more dangerous during wars.

The first response to COVID-19 was quarantine, separating the infected from the well. People were either urged or ordered to stay in their houses, domestic travel was curtailed, and borders were closed. China opted for a draconian quarantine imposed on some 373 million of its residents, many of whom were involuntarily confined without adequate food, water, or sanitation. That quarantine cost the Chinese gross domestic product an estimated $1.7 trillion when cities with populations in the millions were locked down.

Quarantine is expensive, tramples individual freedom, and is the least effective way to stop an epidemic. COVID-19 has taught us how difficult quarantine is and that it is insufficient to stop a pandemic even under the most rigid conditions. That difficulty is multiplied many times over when combatants and refugees are aggregated and moved en masse in wartime. The current war in Ukraine, with the displacement of 10 million internal and external refugees, may yet precipitate epidemics of COVID-19, HIV, hepatitis, and drug-resistant tuberculosis, all of which were endemic in the country before the Russian invasion.

Quarantine aims to control epidemic spread by keeping potential hosts from infecting one another. The second weapon against epidemics is separating the pathogen from potential hosts, and attempts to manipulate the environment to do that came almost simultaneously with quarantine in the COVID-19 epidemic. Food delivered to homes was cleaned before it was brought indoors. Hand sanitizer became ubiquitous as did signs ordering people to stay six feet apart. Mask mandates came and went and came again.

Changing ecology—altering the world in which parasites propagate—dates back as far as quarantine. The earliest recorded sanitary attempts aimed at avoiding fecal contamination of what people ate or drank. The Old Testament directed soldiers to separate latrines from their tents and kitchens and cover them daily with fresh dirt. Pathogens can amplify their range by catching a ride on insects. Flies were associated with sickness in ancient Rome, but the direct connection between insect vectors and contagion was not proven until the nineteenth century. Insect control became part of the armamentarium against epidemics shortly thereafter.

Sanitation remains an integral part of warfare. In the wake of World War I, Hans Zinsser said, "Experience in the cantonments of 1917 and in the sanitation of active troops convincingly showed that war is today, as much as ever, 75 percent an engineering and sanitary problem and a little less than 25 percent a military one. Other things being approximately equal, that army will win which has the best engineering and sanitary services."[1] Late nineteenth-century campaigns against fecal and insect-borne contagion were spectacularly effective, and for a time it looked as if medicine had the upper hand in the fight against epidemics. When I finished medical school in 1970 infectious disease as a specialty was widely considered passé. The serious problems had been solved. COVID-19 has taught us otherwise.

Wars that disrupt and contaminate the ground on which they are fought form a special case of contagion. Attempts to modify the environment to stop the spread of diseases have proven difficult or impossible for armies at war, and that difficulty is magnified manyfold when the disease is airborne and orders of magnitude more by carriers without symptoms.

That said, wars have also given military surgeons unique opportunities to study the ecology of epidemics and have led to innovative ways to control their spread.

The third tool is a case in which the combatant with the best technology and the means to deploy it has an advantage. Pharmacology—drug treatment of infections—has been around for centuries, but until recently there have been very few effective drugs and even fewer that were safe. Mercury is somewhat effective against syphilis and dates to the sixteenth century, but it was also used for a variety of other infections for which it was ineffective. Besides, it is toxic. Chinese physicians used wormwood containing artemisinin, and Jesuit missionaries used cinchona bark and its quinine against malaria at about the same time. Both were effective against malaria but were also used in a broad range of febrile illnesses for which they provided no benefit.

Until the twentieth century those were the only effective treatments for contagious disease, but World War II saw a seismic shift in drug technology. The exigencies of war facilitated pharmacological research that took advantage of the aggregation of large groups of men in controlled situations. The pressure of war expedited trials that might have taken years in peacetime, and a host of stunningly effective antimicrobials came in the mid-twentieth century.

The COVID-19 pandemic has led to the redirection of vast resources intended to develop new antiviral agents. So far those efforts have produced a handful of drugs that ameliorate the disease but few that prevent it and none that cure it. There has also been mistrust of the medical experts who evaluate and approve new treatments, and a variety of speculative and ineffective remedies have captured public attention. Both have occurred in prior wars.

The fourth tool is manipulation of the immune system. Empirical treatments based on the fact that some diseases were caught only once go back hundreds of years. The archetype for immunologic manipulation was smallpox, first with the actual disease and later with *Vaccinia*. As with COVID-19, immunization against smallpox has been controversial, but in military situations it has usually been mandatory, and at least once the result was decisive.

Rather than catalog every war and every epidemic, I have chosen episodes from five American conflicts, each of which illustrates one of the weapons against mass contagion—quarantine, ecology, pharmacology, and immunology—its use or misuse, and how it changed a war's outcome. I have also chosen to tell the stories of the military men (and they were, with rare exception, men) who made difficult decisions with critical results.

We will start with George Washington, the American Revolution, and how smallpox nearly brought the war to an early end. The American Civil War was a story of sequential waves of poorly managed infection, and typhoid in one campaign may well have prolonged the war by three years. The failure to learn from that experience spilled over into the Spanish-American War in which typhoid killed tens of thousands of soldiers who never left the United States. On the positive side a group of young military surgeons conducted a brilliant series of ethically challenged experiments in Cuba that made it possible to live and work in the tropics without dying from yellow fever. During World War I the U.S. Army's failure to quarantine trainees may have caused and certainly facilitated what remains the most lethal pandemic in human history. Finally we will look at the stumbling but ultimately successful pharmacologic control of malaria in World War II. In each case, the epidemic has not gotten the recognition it deserves for its influence on its war, and each case sheds light on the control and controversies surrounding the current pandemic and inevitable future ones.

IMMUNOLOGY

The Virus and the Virginian

D isease in eighteenth-century wars was far more dangerous than battles, and the American Revolution was no exception. It has been estimated that during the Revolution the death rate for American combatants was two hundred of every thousand per year, with only twenty of those deaths caused by battle wounds.[1] Typhus (camp fever) and dysentery were serious problems, but in the war's early years smallpox was the constant, terrifying threat.

SMALLPOX IN HISTORY

Smallpox likely crossed over from domesticated animals in the Nile Valley coincident with the beginnings of agriculture around 10,000 BCE, and it probably spread along trade routes to the riverine cultures of India and China. The mummy of Twentieth Dynasty Pharaoh Rameses V who died in 1157 BCE has pitted scars characteristic of smallpox. There are written descriptions consistent with smallpox from China in 1122 BCE and from India at about the same time. The disease became endemic in Asia and very likely afflicted the army of Alexander the Great when he invaded India.

By 700 CE smallpox had been documented in Japan, Europe, and North Africa. Brought by Spanish conquistadores, it swept through the Western Hemisphere in the sixteenth century. Smallpox was in the Caribbean in 1507, Mexico in 1520, Peru in 1524, and Brazil in 1555. With measles and influenza, it killed 90 percent of the indigenous Incan and Aztec populations in a little over a century. The speed with which smallpox could decimate a population was breathtaking.

In sixteenth-century England, "small pockes" was pervasive. "Pocke," Old English for sac, was a general term for pustules or ulcers, and "small" differentiated the disease from the great pox or syphilis that was raging through Europe at the same time. A year after the arrival of the British "first fleet," the disease devastated Australia's aboriginal population. Smallpox thrived wherever it encountered an immunologically naïve population.

Over the centuries, smallpox has killed more people than any other infectious disease including the Black Plague. In the twentieth century it still killed more than 300 million people. *Variola major*—the severe form that was dominant in the seventeenth and eighteenth centuries—has an approximate 25 percent mortality rate.[2] Eighteenth-century soldier and mathematician Charles-Marie de la Condamine estimated that by his lifetime 10 percent of all mankind had either been killed or disfigured by the disease.[3]

THE ORGANISM

Smallpox is one of a group of pox viruses that includes vaccinia, monkeypox, and a variety of other animal infections. They are the largest animal viruses and overlap the smallest bacteria both in size and complexity, being just visible with very good light microscopes in careful preparations. Their genetic information is carried in a deoxyribonucleic acid (DNA) molecule that is, by viral standards, large and complex as well. The DNA of the smallest viroid has as few as 240 base pairs; smallpox has over 186,000. Human immunodeficiency virus (HIV) forces its host to manufacture 10 viral proteins; smallpox forces 187.

Unlike other DNA viruses, smallpox can co-opt a host cell's cytoplasmic machinery directly without ever entering the nucleus. Two membrane layers (a lipid and a capsomere) surround the hourglass-shaped double-stranded DNA. The result is a $300 \times 250 \times 200$ nanometer brick with rounded corners and a pineapple-skinned knobby surface. In groups smallpox viruses resemble corrugated paving stones.

After the virus enters a host organism it seeks out, adheres to, and penetrates a target cell. Once inside that cell the virus sheds its outer layer and releases its DNA to force the host's cytoplasmic machinery to produce its own messenger ribonucleic acid (mRNA). The pox mRNA makes the host cell produce proteins that further break down the viral core and release viral DNA to both begin replicating and continue the creation of its proteins and more DNA. Those proteins and DNA are assembled into naked viral particles that pick up new external layers. The completed organisms migrate to the host cell's external membrane where about 100,000 new viruses break out of every infected cell to seek out new targets.

THE DISEASE

Some viral particles escape into the environment to find new hosts. Smallpox is transmitted from person to person in two ways. A host might cough an aerosolized particle that can be inhaled and stick to a new host's mucous membranes where it sets off the infectious cascade. Airborne particles can also land on eating or drinking utensils and gain access when they come in contact with a mucous membrane. Smallpox can also spread when fluid oozes from a sore loaded with viruses that persist for weeks in contaminated clothing and bedding.

Smallpox follows a regular and depressingly predictable course. An inhaled virus penetrates cells lining the upper respiratory tract including the mouth and pharynx, and it replicates. The first wave of newly created viruses spills into the bloodstream and spreads to other organs, especially the liver, spleen, and lymph nodes, where they proliferate for ten to twelve days before pouring out in a second viremic flood that causes headache, fever, malaise, generalized aches, sore throat, and a flat red rash.

In the second wave the virus gravitates toward skin and mucous membranes, and vesicles appear in three to four days. The virus also goes wherever there are lining cells that separate the body's interior from the outside world—lungs, kidneys, bladder, intestines, and eyes—and it can be shed in urine, feces, and tears, as well as from pustules. When the intestinal lining is involved a cast of large segments of the bowel wall can be passed. Lips and eyes are sealed shut by the exudate. The tongue and throat swell and make swallowing excruciating. As the disease progresses victims are often unable to talk, but in a cruel irony most remain entirely alert and aware of their suffering. When pustules merge into flat black sheets wide areas of skin and

CHAPTER 1

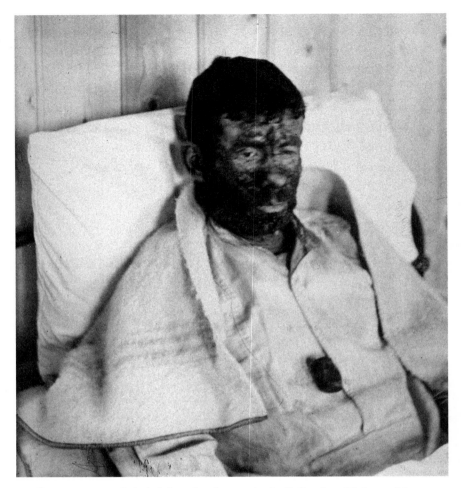

Smallpox was not only lethal, but also devastatingly disfiguring. *Wellcome Library*

mucous membranes simply fall off, and blood oozes from the skin and all orifices. Both the "black" and hemorrhagic forms are almost always fatal.

Overall smallpox mortality is 25–30 percent, and 65–80 percent of survivors are permanently scarred especially on the face. About 1 percent of survivors are blind from viral keratitis or secondary bacterial infection. Modern studies suggest that up to 88 percent of those exposed to the disease contract it, but those numbers are almost all the minor variant of *Variola* that did not exist in the eighteenth century when infectivity and severity were significantly higher.

Pustules last five to eight days before rupturing and crusting over. The smell of smallpox was so strong that it permeated streets and paths around sufferers' homes. The stench came not from decaying flesh but from gas produced in the pustules, and it was said to be distinctive enough that the disease could be diagnosed from a considerable distance. The disease was ugly, lethal, and frightening, and it was a constant presence in colonial America.

SMALLPOX IN THE COLONIES

North America was weeks from European centers of learning, and colonial medical care was rudimentary. In 1775, the colonies had 3,500 medical practitioners, but only 400 had any academic training—350 from universities at Edinburgh, London, Leyden, or Paris, and 50 more from American institutions. The rest were trained by apprenticeship to physicians, surgeons, and apothecaries; Boston had only one university-trained physician. Much of medical knowledge and no small amount of the practice resided with educated laymen, particularly clergy and government officials. In the agrarian southern colonies, medicine was often in the hands of farmers and plantation owners or their wives.

Theories of disease and treatment reflected the practitioners' level of education. Galenic theory held that diseases, rather than being specific entities, were an imbalance of blood, phlegm, black bile, and yellow bile, the body's four humors. The theory led to efforts to restore balance by removing supposed excess humors with purgatives, emetics, and bleeding. Those therapies persisted well into the nineteenth century, and they were directly related to Sir William Osler's contention that it was nearly 1900 before a patient could visit a doctor and have a statistical likelihood of profiting from the encounter.

Folk remedies were based on repelling evil influences with noxious substances that might have been harvested from toads, vermin, or feces. Indian cures derived from local plants and animals were common as well. In the eighteenth century, there were only two drugs effective for specific indications. Cinchona was used for malaria but also for other fevers for which it was useless. Mercury was known to be effective against syphilis, but it was too dangerous for regular use. There was nothing for smallpox.

Physicians and laymen knew some diseases came in outbreaks, and the miasmic theory of contagion held that a combination of the decomposition of organic matter coupled with adverse changes in the climate or atmosphere caused those diseases. Yellow fever, malaria, and plague were classed as miasmic until the nineteenth century when pathogenic microbes and their insect vectors were identified. Exanthems were not blamed on miasms; it was obvious that measles and smallpox could pass from person to person.

For the most part the colonies contributed little to medical science. The first medical publication in North America, Thomas Thacher's *Brief Rule to Guide the Common People of New England How to Order Themselves and Theirs in the Small Pocks or Measles*, was just an uncredited rehash of material previously published in England by Thomas Sydenham.

Smallpox was in the colonies from their beginning. The disease came to New England before the Puritan settlers and played a major role in their early survival. Between 1617 and 1619 an epidemic brought by English traders wiped out 90 percent of Massachusetts' indigenous population leaving unoccupied, cultivated fields that fed the Pilgrim settlers when they arrived two seasons later. In 1677 and 1678, ships from England repeatedly brought smallpox to colonial seaports. (Thacher's pamphlet was written in September 1678 after 150 people had died of the disease in Boston.)

New England epidemics recurred in 1690, 1702–3, and 1721. The last coincided with an outbreak in London that resulted in an effective way to control the disease. Prior to 1721, sanitation and quarantine were all that was available to manage smallpox. Patients' clothes and bedding were aired out or burned, and ships' holds and their cargos were decontaminated with smoke. In 1718, the Massachusetts General Court built a quarantine facility on Spectacle Island where every ship with passengers or crew suspected of having smallpox was held until certified healthy. When the 1721 Boston epidemic peaked, the selectmen either removed the infected to a pest house or placed red flags on their homes, fenced their houses off, and placed guards around them, but quarantine was far from foolproof. When HMS *Seahorse* arrived in Boston its master took his sick Negro servant ashore and precipitated the outbreak that infected 5,980 of the city's 10,670 residents and killed 844 of them. Most Bostonians fled the city, and only about seven hundred of those who stayed and were not immune from having previously had the disease escaped smallpox.[4]

The disease was general in England as well. Between 1731 and 1765 the London Bills of Mortality listed an average of 23,300 deaths a year, 9 percent of which were from smallpox. Between 1675 and 1775 smallpox was absent from the colonies for as long as five years only twice.[5] In North America, port cities were most at risk with Boston and Charleston the worst followed closely by New York and Philadelphia. The disease periodically reappeared throughout the colonies; it reduced populations, generated quarantine restrictions, and ruined economies.

INOCULATION

All that changed after 1721. It had long been known that one never got smallpox twice, and that was used to advantage in Asia. Inoculation involved deliberately giving previously uninfected people smallpox to create lifelong immunity, and manipulating the immune system was demonstrably more effective than sanitation and quarantine. It is important to understand that inoculation was different from the vaccination that came at the end of the eighteenth century. Vaccination uses a virus similar to one that causes clinical smallpox but rarely causes systemic disease. Inoculation is purposely giving the patient the actual disease under controlled circumstances; those inoculated are both at risk from the disease and contagious to those around them.

Since the tenth century Chinese physicians had collected the dried crust from smallpox lesions, saved it as a powder, and used a straw to blow it up noses to create controlled disease. The Persians did the same but administered the powder by mouth where it entered the body through the mucous membranes. In India the powder was injected under the skin. Data on the risk and effectiveness of those inoculations are unavailable, but it is unlikely the practice would have persisted for centuries if inoculation with smallpox-contaminated matter had not been less dangerous than catching the disease naturally.

Why did inoculation create a less lethal disease? Cotton Mather, minister of Boston's Calvinist North Church, suggested that injecting smallpox-containing matter into a limb far from the body's vital organs was safer than acquiring it naturally since the disease had farther to travel. Perhaps injected matter was safer than an inhaled aerosol. Mather also suggested that the injected pox used up the body's supply of fuel leaving the wild virus starved and unable to cause disease. It is more likely that the virus was weakened by harvesting and processing before it was put in the body, less virulent but still able to generate immunity, or the matter may have been intentionally taken from patients with less severe illness. No one has intentionally used inoculation for over two hundred years, so we can only guess why it caused less disease than smallpox acquired in the "natural way."

Rumors of inoculation had reached London as early as 1700 when Martin Lister reported hearing about it from a relative who had traveled to China. Clopton Havers reported on the practice in a communication to the Royal Society where it was again discussed in 1713 and 1714. In 1716 Emanuel Timon, who had been born in Greece and studied medicine in Padua and at Oxford, published "An Account, or History, of Procuring the SMALLPOX by Incision or Inoculation; as It Has for Some Time Been Practised at Constantinople" in the *Philosophical Transactions of the Royal Society*. A similar report came from Jacobus Pylarini of Venice, but neither resulted in general use of the procedure. That was left to Lady Mary Wortley Montagu who had accompanied her husband to Constantinople when he was Great Britain's ambassador to the Sublime Porte. She had been a great beauty before smallpox permanently scarred her, so her interest in inoculation was personal. When Lady Mary returned to London in 1721 smallpox was rampant, and she resolved to do something about it. She inoculated seven convicts, eleven underaged paupers, and her own two children. Two of the twenty died, and the procedure was temporarily discredited, but even a 10 percent death rate was less than that of the natural disease, and many of London's well-to-do adopted the procedure.[6]

INOCULATION IN THE COLONIES

Inoculation spread across the Atlantic almost immediately and became the American colonies' most important contribution to medical science. Cotton Mather was arguably the best educated and most widely read man in the city. The son and grandson of three of Boston's most prominent

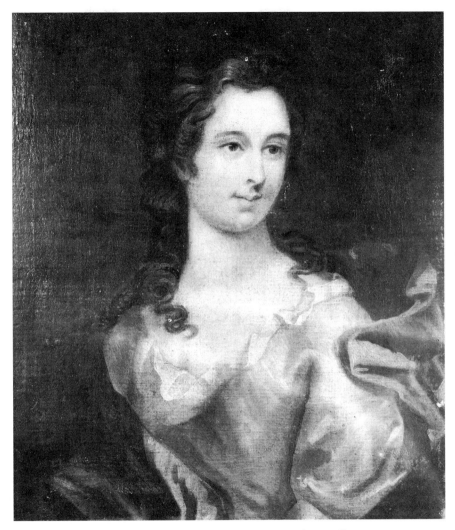

Lady Mary Wortley Montague introduced inoculation for smallpox to Western medicine. *Wellcome Library*

ministers, Mather attended Boston Latin School and graduated from Harvard at age fifteen. He nearly gave up on following his forbears into the ministry because a severe speech impediment rendered him virtually unable to speak in public. As an alternative to preaching he concentrated on medicine while working to control the stuttering. Practice helped his speech, and Mather was ordained in 1685, but his interest in medicine persisted. He started writing letters to the Royal Society in 1712 and penned more than a hundred unpublished short scientific reports over the next dozen years.

In 1716, Mather wrote London physician John Woodward describing a conversation he had with his Negro slave Onesimus.[7] When he asked the slave if he had had smallpox in Africa, Onesimus said he had "something of the disease," and he described being inoculated before being captured. Mather heard a similar story from other Boston slaves who reported having gotten a mild disease with ten to thirty pustules that protected them for the rest of their lives. Mather told the story to Reverend Benjamin Colman who confirmed the practice with more slaves and those who traded them.

In 1720 Mather collected his thoughts on medicine into a pamphlet, *The Angel of Bethesda*, in which science was liberally mixed with religion including the contention that disease was divine punishment for original sin. Smallpox, being especially loathsome, was special punishment and worthy of particular shame. For all that Mather presaged the germ theory of disease more than a century and a half before it was widely accepted. Referring to the microscopist Anton van Leuwenhoek's animalcules, he wondered if "one species of these Animals may offend in one way and another in another, and various parts may be offended: from whence may flow a Variety of Diseases."[8] The pamphlet never garnered enough subscribers to be published, and Mather's ideas lay fallow. The manuscript was held uncatalogued and unrecognized by the American Antiquarian Society until it was rediscovered and printed in 1972.

William Douglass, Boston's one university-trained physician, loaned Mather a copy of the *Philosophical Transactions* that described intentional inoculation in Asia, and the minister was reminded of Onesimus' story. When a Boston epidemic broke out Mather wondered how many lives might be saved if it were practiced.[9] His attempts to get Boston practitioners to try inoculation, however, caused an uproar. Douglass was angry that a layman would intrude into medicine. Besides, how could one justify intentionally giving a healthy person a lethal disease? In addition an inoculated person would be infectious and would almost certainly spread the disease. Finally—and perhaps most persuasively in Calvinist Boston—inoculation

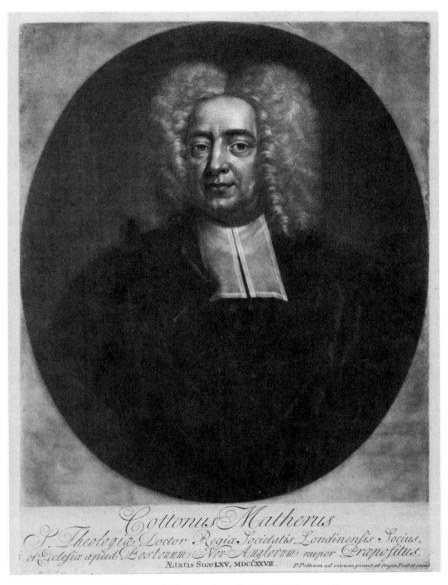

Cottonus Matherus

S. Theologiæ Doctor Regiæ Societatis Londinensis Socius, et Ecclesiæ apud Bostonum Nov Anglorum nuper Præpositus.

Ætatis Suæ LXV, MDCCXXVII. P. Pelham ad vivum pinxit ab Origin Fecit et excud.

Cotton Mather brought inoculation to the colonies. *Wellcome Library*

was a clear interference with God's will. Arguments against immunization are not peculiar to twenty-first-century epidemics.

The only physician Mather could convince to try inoculation was Zabdiel Boylston, owner of the largest apothecary shop in South Boston. He verified Mather's Onesimus story, and on June 26, 1721, he inoculated two of his slaves and his thirteen-year-old son. Boylston did not inoculate himself since he had had the disease and assumed he was immune. He injected matter from smallpox pustules into the arms, legs, and neck of his subjects, covered the areas with walnut shells to keep them from being scratched, and waited.

His son developed more than one hundred pustules and became quite ill. Although the boy survived, Boylston was arrested for having inoculated him and was forced to hide in his house during the day for two weeks; he could safely make house calls only after dark and in disguise. Nevertheless, Boylston inoculated another ten people by July 17. He did seventeen more in August, thirty-one in September, eighteen in October, and more than one hundred in November. Almost all were of Boston's upper class who could afford the complicated procedure, a fact particularly galling to the egalitarian Douglass.

In November a "granado" was thrown through Mather's front window with a note: "COTTON MATHER, You dog, Dam you, I'll inoculate you with this, with a Pox to you."[10] The furor, however, subsided with the epidemic. By May it was over, but Boylston continued inoculating, now with the specific permission of Boston's selectmen. The government licensed a medical procedure for the first time in the colonies, and the course of smallpox in New England permanently changed.

Boylston went on to inoculate 248 people, and he and Mather kept detailed records of who was treated and their outcome. In his report to the Royal Society (*Historical Account of the Small-Pox Inoculated in New England*) he noted that one of six Bostonians who had smallpox "in the natural way" died. For those inoculated it was only one in sixty. Boylston's was the first quantitative medical study in North America and one of the first in the world. His report led to the resumption of widespread inoculation in London where a study of more than one thousand cases showed a 16.6 percent mortality from natural smallpox and only 2 percent from inoculation. When the procedure spread from England to Europe the Americans were specifically credited, and Mather was elected fellow of the Royal Society in 1726. The controversy was, however, far from over. James Franklin's *New England Courant* (where his brother Benjamin was an apprentice) aggressively attacked both Boylston and Mather.[11] The selectmen thought better of their permission, reprimanded Boylston, and ordered him to cease inoculations. He refused.

When the disease returned in 1729 local citizens petitioned the selectmen to again allow inoculation. That year 400 Bostonians were inoculated of whom 12 died (3 percent). Among 3,600 natural cases, there were 500 deaths (14 percent).[12] The numbers in the next outbreak in 1751 were even more striking. Out of a population of 15,684, half were either immune or left the city. Of the non-immunes who stayed, 5,545 caught smallpox and 539 (almost 10 percent) died. Of the 2,124 who were inoculated only 30 died (1.4 percent).[13]

In New England acceptance of inoculation spread, and by 1764 smallpox in New England was almost always brought from other colonies. That year there were 894 deaths from smallpox in New England while only 46 who had been inoculated died.[14] If one tracks the rate of inoculation in Boston through the epidemics the numbers are even more impressive. In 1721 Boylston and Mather managed to inoculate only 2 percent of the population. In 1730 that rose to 10 percent, 28 percent in 1752, and 87 percent in 1764.

The procedure was never cheap. In 1764 it cost one pound, five shillings, four pence for medications and personal attendance as well as three dollars a week for food, nursing, and "necessities." That did not count the six weeks of lost income during recovery.

A variety of inoculation methods were employed in England and the colonies. The earliest was "Boerhavian" and emphasized rigorous preparation for several weeks before inoculation in an attempt to regulate the body so it would be ready to accept the disease. The inoculators wanted what they called an entire alteration of the blood and juices to get the patient safely through the ordeal to come. Preparation included the administration of thirty to forty grains of mercury to induce salivation and purging two to three times a day. Meat and broth were to be avoided during preparation and after the procedure. After inoculation the patient was kept at bed rest and wrapped in blankets to sweat out the disease.

London physician Robert Sutton modified the procedure to make it less onerous. He used Sydenham's "cool method" rather than sweating and abandoned the preparation period. When possible Sutton obtained material for inoculation from another inoculee that may have resulted in the reuse of an attenuated form of the virus. He took only clear inoculum, avoided lesions that had suppurated, and injected in a cut only deep enough to draw a drop of blood. He also quarantined those inoculated to avoid spreading the disease.[15] Sutton tried to keep the details of his procedure secret, but Thomas Dimsdale had learned the method and published a pamphlet describing it in 1767. Dimsdale's pamphlet was reprinted in New York in 1771, and variations of the Dimsdale method were standard in the colonies, although two weeks of light, meat-free diet, and doses of calomel and antimony and occasional purging were still employed.

Legal control of inoculation varied from colony to colony and from decade to decade. A Boston pamphlet in 1721 suggested that if any patient died from inoculation the inoculator should be hanged. There were a variety of less radical attempts to regulate the practice especially to protect non-immunes from being infected by those inoculated. Boston allowed the procedure whenever at least twenty local families had smallpox as long as approval from the selectmen was obtained. Connecticut and Rhode Island banned the procedure outright. New York issued an executive proclamation in 1747, "strictly prohibiting and forbidding all and every of the Doctors, Physicians, Surgeons, and Practitioners of Physick, and all and every other persons within this Province, to inoculate for smallpox any persons or person within the City and County of New York, on pain of being prosecuted to the utmost rigour of the law."[16] A 1738 law in Charleston levied a £500 fine on anyone found to have inoculated within two miles of the city. When an outbreak became general, attitudes abruptly changed. For a time during the 1764 Boston epidemic anyone who wished could be inoculated.

A decisive factor in spreading the practice in Boston was the agreement by the town's physicians to treat the poor for free. A combination of public acceptance and free care made the practice general during outbreaks, and people flooded into the city seeking inoculation. The selectmen warned that the town was becoming one large inoculation hospital, and the General Court levied fines for anyone who came to Boston to be inoculated and added penalties for breaking quarantine after the procedure. During one epidemic it was made illegal to communicate the disease either intentionally or by accident, effectively making it against the law to contract smallpox either naturally or by inoculation.

Between outbreaks public acceptance of inoculation waned. Citizens fearful of being infected by inoculated patients convinced the General Court to close an inoculation hospital on Nantucket Island in 1771, and another such facility in Marblehead was burned by arsonists in 1773. In 1775 Boston banned all inoculation, but that ban was short-lived.

In July 1776 smallpox broke out in Boston along with the spreading Revolutionary War and the resulting movement of troops, and the ban was suspended. Harvard delayed commencement so the entire senior class could be inoculated along with almost five thousand other Bostonians. Only those certified as free of smallpox were allowed to leave the city, and only those known to be immune were allowed in. The combination of quarantine and inoculation worked; by August 22 there were only seventy-eight cases in the city. By September 14 there were only eighteen; the quarantine was lifted, and inoculation was again restricted. In April 1777, the General Court ordered that government permission be obtained before opening an inoculation hospital. If permission was granted each patient had to post a £10 bond and each physician one of £500 to guarantee that quarantine would be enforced during the contagious period after inoculation.

Virginia was more rigid. A 1769 act mandated an astronomical £1,000 fine for anyone who imported "any variolous or infectious matter" for inoculation. Civil authorities could license inoculation on a limited basis, but there was a £100 fine for inoculating without that license.

The 1769 Act was later rewritten by a committee comprising George Mason, Richard Lee, and Thomas Jefferson, but Jefferson still had to go to Philadelphia to be inoculated since the procedure remained prohibitively inconvenient in Virginia. Before a household could be inoculated permission had to be obtained from every other household within a two-mile radius unless separated by a river or creek at least half a mile wide. After inoculation the patient had to either remain at home or warn anyone he encountered until entirely free of infection. The inoculating physician had to place a warning on the nearest road or "other notorious place" advising

that smallpox was present. There was a 40 shilling per day fine for not posting such a sign and a £500 fine or six months in jail for violating the law.[17]

Pennsylvania and to a lesser extent New Jersey, Maryland, and rural
New York were more liberal. Pennsylvania allowed inoculation without
any restriction save for a single quarantine law that was seldom enforced.
Pennsylvania and the others advertised inoculation hospital services
in New England and the southern colonies. Abigail Adams traveled to
Philadelphia from her home in Quincy, Massachusetts, to be inoculated
although she continued a lively social life during a recovery in which she
was surely contagious.

By 1775 the medical profession and probably the majority of the public
were convinced that inoculation, while risky for those receiving it as well as
those exposed to them, was less dangerous than naturally occurring smallpox. The compromise was to limit the procedure when the disease was not
prevalent and to loosen those restrictions when it was.

SMALLPOX AND THE REVOLUTION

George Washington was a provincial planter of modest estate and questionable military ability when he was given command of the "Army of the
United Colonies" (the Continental Army) by the Second Continental Congress on June 15, 1775. His subsequent accomplishments as commander of
the Continental Army and as the nation's first chief executive earned him
a unique position in history. What is less well known is that he ordered
the first wartime immunization of an entire army. Without that order the
Revolution would likely have failed.

Washington was physically imposing; at six feet, two inches, he was
six inches taller than the average eighteenth-century American man. He
weighed about 175 pounds as a young man with more of that weight in his
hips and thighs than in his arms and chest. His 1772 Charles Wilson Peale
portrait from life is quite unlike the nineteenth-century one Horatio Greenough did from imagination and reputation that shows a middle-aged head
grafted onto a bodybuilder's torso. The contemporary image shows rather
narrow shoulders and a waist straining the buttons of a stretched waistcoat.
That said, those who described him in life were remarkably consistent in
praising his grace, athleticism, and presence. Philadelphia physician and

signer of the Declaration of Independence Benjamin Rush told his friend Thomas Ruston that Washington would make any of Europe's kings look like a valet de chambre.

Washington attended the first Continental Congress in 1774 as a delegate from Virginia, but when the Congress convened for a second time the

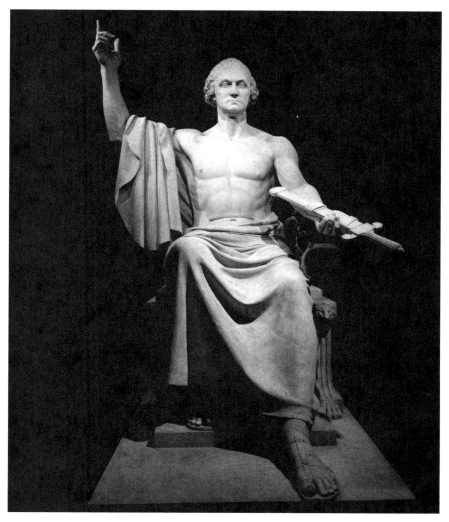

Horace Greenough's fanciful statue of George Washington, who ordered all Continental troops to be inoculated during the American Revolution. *Smithsonian Institution*

following year he came with a different outfit and a different role. Unlike the other frock-coated delegates, the Virginian wore the blue and buff uniform he had designed for the Fairfax County militia. He sported an impressive array of brass buttons but no mark of rank. When Washington took command in Boston he had to buy a ribbon for his coat so the men would recognize him. He planned to leave the Philadelphia congress as a soldier, but he expected to command Virginia's forces and not an entire army.

There were certainly other candidates to lead the colonies' military effort. Charles Lee had been an officer in the British Army and had fought in the French and Indian War. He reached the rank of major general in the Polish Army and fought with the Russians against the Ottoman Empire before buying a Virginia farm in 1773. Lee was brash and uncouth, and he had more military experience than anyone else in the colonies.[18] Wealthy New York landowner and businessman Philip Schuyler had also served in the French and Indian War as had Massachusetts native Israel Putnam.[19] "Old Put" had fought with Rogers' Rangers, had barely escaped being burned alive after being captured by Mohawk Indians, and was adored by the men who had fought with him at Bunker Hill. All three, along with Artemas Ward who was in command at Boston, were made major generals.

Although Washington thought that declining command would be a stain on his honor and a disappointment to his friends, he had serious misgivings: "Lest some unlucky event should happen unfavorable to my reputation, I beg it may be remembered, by every gentleman in the room, that I declare with the utmost sincerity, I do not think myself equal to the command I am honored with."[20] He went on to warn Congress that "my Abilities and Military experience may not be equal to the extensive and important trust" they placed in him.[21] He delayed telling his wife who expected him back at Mount Vernon as soon as the Congress adjourned, and when he did tell her he swore that he had made every effort to avoid the appointment.

Washington had several qualifications for command in the eyes of the delegates. First he was from Virginia. Members from outside New England were acutely aware that the war had started in Massachusetts, and the northern colonies had raised the first armies and named the first generals.

There was real concern that the New England colonies would dominate any revolution and would keep that dominance in the event of a successful outcome. Besides—and this was a factor that would come back in 1782—Washington's apparent hesitance to assume so much power was reassuring. Altogether, Congress was pleased to send him to take command in Boston.

BOSTON

The geography of Boston changed after the Back Bay was filled in beginning in 1857, but in 1775 the town sat on an irregular mushroom of land connected to the mainland by a narrow neck pointed south toward Roxbury. On the northwest the city was separated from Charlestown by a narrow passage between the harbor and the mouth of the Charles River. North of Charlestown were Breed's Hill and Bunker Hill on a peninsula recently taken by the British and connected to the mainland by a narrow neck pointed northwest. A third peninsula containing Dorchester Heights looked down on the city from the southeast. British forces were concentrated in Boston with a few in Charlestown and a few more occupying the connection between the town and the mainland north of Roxbury. The Continentals had headquarters at Roxbury and up the Charles River at Cambridge. Their forces were in a ring extending from northwest of Charlestown all the way around to Dorchester, but the British could be resupplied by sea, and a direct assault on the town would either have to come from the bay or go across the narrow neck from Roxbury. On the other hand the hills around Dorchester looked straight down on the Commons where most of the British were camped.

In early July the new commanding general took a small carriage from Philadelphia through New York to Watertown, Massachusetts, where the colony's congress was meeting. They were only three miles from the Continental Army's camp at Cambridge across the Charles River from Boston. Washington and the other new generals quietly slipped into the camp to an uncertain welcome; Ward and most of his soldiers saw the imposition of the Virginian as an insult.

What Washington found in Cambridge was not what he had been led to expect. He had been told there were 10,000 to 12,000 British regulars in Boston, and he estimated that it would take at least twice that many untrained militias to dislodge them. Before leaving Philadelphia he had been told he had 20,000 men in Boston, and one of his first acts as commander-in-chief was to ask his unit commanders for an exact count. Their delay in responding confirmed that all was not as it had been presented. Washington eventually found he had about 16,000 men, only 14,000 of whom were healthy. Dysentery and camp fever (typhus) were rife, and smallpox was enough of a threat that the Massachusetts provisional congress had already established a quarantine hospital in anticipation of an outbreak.

Numbers were not Washington's only problem. The new commander was impressed with neither the New England private soldiers nor their officers. He wrote his cousin Lund Washington that the officers were, "generally speaking the most indifferent kind of people I ever saw." The men "would fight very well if properly officered, although they are an exceedingly dirty and nasty people."[22] He complained about "an unaccountable kind of stupidity in the lower classes of these people" that spilled over "too generally among the officers of the Massachusetts part of the army who are nearly all of the same kidney with the privates."[23]

The problem came in large part from New England's egalitarian democracy. The officers were mostly elected by their men, and they did not see their station as separate from them—if the officers had been barbers before enlisting they continued to cut the men's hair afterward. The regiments operated as semi-autonomous clubs.

Washington and Lee set out to separate the men from the officers, issued consistent daily orders from regiment to regiment, and started to clean up the camps. The New Englanders were farmers and mechanics, not professional soldiers. On the one hand, they had built reasonably good shelters, many of wood and some with actual doors and windows. On the other hand, they were from widely separated rural communities and had no experience living in close quarters. Sanitation was abysmal. The men saw no reason to dig "necessaries," and the whole place stank. Two days after the new generals arrived from Philadelphia they ordered line officers to see that their men were neat and clean and that the "necessaries" were taken care of. And no one was allowed to fish in Fresh Pond where the smallpox hospital had been built.

Smallpox was more than a potential threat. In the summer of 1775 Boston started one of its periodic epidemics. There had not been a serious outbreak in over a decade, so a considerable part of the present population was not immune. British commander Sir William Howe ordered that every one of his occupying troops and all their families be inoculated unless they were demonstrably immune. Inoculations put the non-immune civilian population at risk, and by July most Bostonians who could afford it had fled. Just over 6,500 tradesmen, artisans, and paupers were left.[24]

Howe had a significant advantage since most of his troops were immune either from inoculation or from having had smallpox as children. If the disease broke out among Boston civilians it posed a greater threat to the Continentals than to his army. Smallpox was, in effect, a weapon Howe had that Washington did not.

Washington needed to act since most of his New Englanders served under contracts due to expire at the end of 1775, and if they left it would mean recruiting, clothing, and training a whole new army. Even if he had the manpower to attack Boston, doing so with an army susceptible to smallpox would almost certainly have been a disaster.

Washington had more than abstract knowledge of smallpox. In 1751, at age nineteen, he went to Barbados with his brother Lawrence, who was looking for a climate to help his worsening consumption. The two Virginians landed at Bridgetown on November 2, and two weeks later George had the first symptoms of smallpox. Details of the illness are lacking because Washington put no entries into his diary for the next few weeks, but it was probably a relatively mild case, and it left only a few scars on his nose. Barbados did not work out well for Lawrence, and he went on to Bermuda looking for a better climate while George returned to Mount Vernon. Lawrence finally came home on July 26 and died of tuberculosis shortly thereafter.[25]

Fear of smallpox kept the Continentals out of Boston, geography penned the British inside the city, and civilians were dying in an epidemic. The citizens petitioned the Massachusetts legislature to let them leave if the British would allow it, but Washington was not enthusiastic. He was convinced that an epidemic spread by civilians would destroy his army, and he was unwilling to take his entire force out of commission for the month necessary to inoculate the men. A few civilians were allowed to take ferries to Salem or Chelsea where they could be quarantined, but even that was stopped early in October. In a November 28 general order Washington banned all refugees from his camps and ordered that all correspondence from Boston be dipped in vinegar to be disinfected before being opened.

Fear of smallpox was compounded by the suspicion that the British were using the disease as a weapon. Rumors spread that Howe was inoculating refugees before letting them leave the city. Robert Harrison, Washington's aide-de-camp, wrote the Council of Massachusetts on December 3, "Four deserters have just arrived at headquarters giving an account that several persons are to be sent out of Boston . . . that have lately been inoculated with the smallpox, with the design, probably to spread infection to distress us as much as possible."[26] The rumor was verified separately in a letter from Colonel Loammi Baldwin who called it an "unheard of diabolical scheme."[27] The following day Washington wrote John Hancock, "By recent information from Boston, Genl. Howe is going to send out a number of Inhabitants in order it is thought to make more room for his expected reinforcements, there is one part of the information that I can hardly give Credibility. A sailor says that a number of these coming out have been inoculated, with design of spreading the smallpox thro' this Country and Camps. I have communicated this to the General Court & recommended their attention thereto."[28] An addendum to the note added that three hundred refugees had recently arrived at Point Shirley. The rumors were spreading and the threat was real, but Washington could not bring himself to believe that the British would stoop to using disease as a weapon of war.

A week later, he changed his mind. Again to Hancock: "The information I received that the enemy intended spreading the smallpox amongst us I would not suppose them capable of. I now must give some credit to it, as it has made its appearance on several of those who last came out of Boston, every necessary precaution has been taken to prevent its being communicated to this Army, & the General Court will take Care, that it does not Spread through the Country."[29] The General Court ordered that anyone coming out of Boston be held at Point Shirley long enough to be proven free of disease and to have all of their clothing and personal effects smoked and disinfected.

Howe had made Boston difficult to invade by allowing smallpox to spread among the civilians, and now he appeared to be using it as an offensive weapon as well. On December 15, Washington wrote Lieutenant Colonel Joseph Reed, "The Smallpox is in every part of Boston—the soldiers there who have never had it, are we are told under Inoculation—& consider'd as a Security against any attempt of ours. A third ship load of People is come out to Point Shirley—If we escape the Smallpox in this Camp, & in the Country round about it, it will be miraculous—Every precaution that can be is taken to guard against this Evil both by the General Court and myself."[30]

On March 17, 1776, Washington stole a march on the British and moved cannons captured from the British at Fort Ticonderoga to Dorchester Heights and made Boston untenable for the British. Howe ordered the city evacuated, and eight thousand troops and followers and one thousand Tory sympathizers boarded ships and sailed for Halifax on March 22.

That did not solve Washington's smallpox problem. He was convinced that "the Smallpox is in every part of Boston," and he was equally sure it was an intentional strategy to infect the Continental Army.[31] When the British left he sorted through his army to find one thousand soldiers with smallpox scars to accompany him into Boston, and he gave strict orders that no one else enter the city. The general "expressly orders, that neither Officer, or Soldier, presume to go into Boston, without leave from General in Chief at Cambridge, or commanding general at Roxbury" since "the enemy with a malicious assiduity, have spread the infection of the smallpox through all parts of the town."[32] On April 14, Washington left two regiments under Ward to guard the city and departed for New York City where he expected Howe to attack. He was correct. Howe and his troops sailed from Halifax and arrived in New York in June.

Through July the epidemic raged. Inoculation had been banned in the Army to avoid spreading the disease, but the ban was lifted for twelve days that month, and Ward arranged to have his non-immune troops inoculated. Almost five thousand Massachusetts citizens "took the pox" as well.

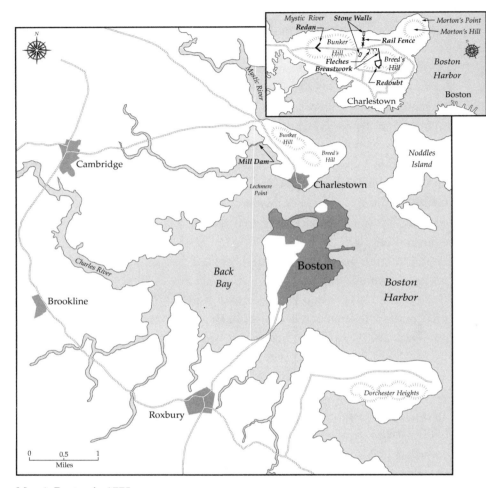

Map 1. Boston in 1775

Only those without smallpox were allowed to leave Boston, and only those who were immune were allowed to enter. It was a mandate with teeth, and the combination of quarantine and immunization ended the epidemic. By the end of August there were only seventy-eight cases. By mid-September there were eighteen, and the quarantine was lifted. Altogether in 1776 there were 5,292 cases of smallpox in Boston, but 4,988 were from inoculation and there were only twenty-eight deaths.[33]

Even though Boston was no longer a problem for Washington, small-pox very much was. Besides the direct threat of an outbreak, fear of disease was making recruiting difficult. Worried about flagging enlistment from Virginia, Washington's brother wrote, "I know the danger of the smallpox and camp fever is more alarming to many than any danger they apprehend from the arms of the enemy."[34] Disease and diminishing numbers of new recruits threatened to render the Northern Army useless. Washington had managed smallpox in Boston with quarantine, but it was obvious that more had to be done to keep the Continental Army functional and the problem was about to get worse.

CANADA

Early in the war the Continentals harbored the reasonable assumption that French Canadians, only twelve years from being conquered by the British, would look favorably on a revolt against the British crown. They might be willing or even anxious to participate. Lake Champlain, Lake George, and the Hudson River were loosely linked into a navigable route by which Canada could be invaded. Conversely the British could use the lakes and river to carve New England off from the rest of the colonies.

The invasion plan had two prongs. Philip Schuyler was meant to lead one army across the lakes to the Richelieu River and into Canada, but rheumatism and an attack of scurvy prevented his staying with the invasion, so Brig. Gen. Richard Montgomery replaced him in September. Montgomery was an Ulster Scots Irishman who had fought as a British regular in the French and Indian War including a campaign in western New York and the Lakes after which he moved to New York, became a farmer, and married an American. In May 1775 he was elected to the New York Provincial Congress, and a month later was commissioned brigadier general in the Continental Army.[35]

Montgomery's force left Crown Point at the southern end of Lake Champlain on August 28 with 1,500 men from Massachusetts, Connecticut, and New York and trekked to Fort St. John, which guarded Montreal from the south. By the time he got to the fort, 937 of Montgomery's men had to be discharged for illness. He received two thousand replacements and took the fort on November 3.[36] Montreal capitulated without opposition on November 13 after British commander General Guy Carleton and his troops sailed down the St. Lawrence to Quebec City.

The second invasion under Col. Benedict Arnold proceeded from the Maine coast up the Kennebec River to the Chaudière River and on to the St. Lawrence and Quebec City. On September 11, Arnold set out with 1,100 men from Pennsylvania, Maryland, Virginia, and New England and with an abysmal ignorance of Maine geography. He thought it was 180 miles from the coast to Quebec; it was twice that. He also assumed that the Kennebec would be mostly navigable with only a handful of short portages, but the river had long rapids that swamped and capsized his four-hundred-pound boats. The bateaux had been hastily built of green pine, and besides being massive they were porous and barely floated. Salt cod, the expedition's main source of protein, lay uncovered in the bottom of the boats where fresh water rinsed out the salt, and the fish rotted. Provision barrels soaked through, and the bread in them swelled and burst the containers. The men were reduced to half rations of wet flour and spoiled salt pork.

The portage between the Kennebec and the Chaudière Rivers was a nightmare. The men carried the boats, supplies, and equipment in mud up to their knees for three days looking for the Chaudière. "In this state of uncertainty we wandered through hideous swamps and mountainous precipices, with the conjoint addition of cold, wet and hunger, not to mention our fatigue—with the terrible apprehension of famishing in this desert."[37] The men were forced to eat whatever came to hand: shaving soap, lip balm, shoe leather, cartridge boxes, and the company dog.[38] By mid-October Arnold's force was down to 950 effectives, and 300 of those quit and went home. What was left of the army arrived outside Quebec on December 2 starving, frostbitten, and without most of their equipment. They had no field pieces, no bayonets, and only four rounds of ammunition per man.[39]

To make a dire situation worse, Quebec was in the midst of a smallpox outbreak that had started the previous month, and Arnold's exhausted men were easy victims. Smallpox appeared in the American force on December 8. At first it was not widespread; by the eighteenth only five cases were hospitalized, and those were likely from Americans' interaction with local inhabitants although Arnold's men suspected that the British had deliberately sent diseased Quebecois to infect them. As in Boston, the British soldiers were largely immune while the Continentals were not. What started as sporadic infections became an epidemic, and by the end of the month

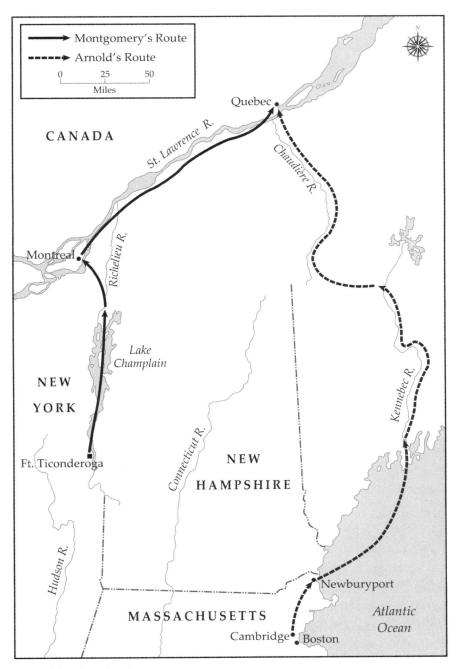

Map 2. The Canadian Invasion

there were two hundred cases among the Americans. The New Englanders knew about smallpox epidemics, and both officers and men started inoculating themselves despite specific orders to the contrary.

Meanwhile, Montgomery left a small force at Montreal and sent three hundred troops on to Quebec. There was real urgency because most of those men's enlistments were due to end on January 1, and out of fear of smallpox most refused to reenlist.

Convinced he had to act, Montgomery attacked Quebec City the night of December 31. The attack was a disaster. The Americans lost fifty-four men including Montgomery, and the survivors settled into a prolonged, ineffective siege.

Smallpox almost immediately broke out among the four hundred soldiers taken prisoner in the failed attack. Sixteen of the thirty-four captured officers paid to have themselves inoculated, but the enlisted men who could not pay died in droves.[40] Private Simon Forbes wrote, "When the pock was coming out in 70–80 of our number, a fever very high and no water to drink, the men drank their own urine which made the fever rage to violently to be endured. Our flesh seemed a mass of corruption. At the same time, we were covered with vermin. When we were a little recovered, we were moved back to our former prison without any cleansing or changing of our apparel. Our clothing was stiff with corrupted matter."[41]

Things were little better for those who had escaped and continued the siege. On February 15, Arnold wrote Washington that he had one hundred men in the hospital, but that number was almost certainly understated. Reinforcements were sent, but most were not immune and promptly took sick. Schuyler, still technically in command though still in New York, told Washington the reinforcements were actually making his army weaker. By the end of March the 2,505 Continentals outside Quebec included 786 too sick to report for duty. By May reinforcements brought the total to 3,200, but 1,200 were sick, mostly from smallpox.[42] John Adams wrote, "The smallpox is ten times more terrible than Britons, Canadians, and Indians together."[43] The Americans in Canada had one of the highest incidences of smallpox of any population in eighteenth-century America.[44] Surgeon Samuel Springer wrote Washington that the army was in a fair way to succumb to smallpox, and there was nothing he could do about it.

On May 10, British reinforcements came up the St. Lawrence, and the Continentals were forced to abandon the siege. Arnold left between two hundred and five hundred men, almost all of whom had smallpox, to be collected by Carleton as he fell back to the trading village of Sorel where the Richelieu emptied into the St. Lawrence.

Brig. Gen. John Thomas, a notoriously difficult man, assumed command. Thomas was a physician who had apprenticed under his father, a British regimental surgeon, and had been doing surgery since he was eighteen years old. He left medicine to take a lieutenant's commission in the British Army in 1747, joined the Massachusetts regiment of volunteers in 1775 as a colonel, and was promoted brigadier general in June of the same year.

Thomas' New Englanders knew inoculation would protect them, and if regimental surgeons would not do it they did it themselves. Thomas did not want men out of commission for weeks while under inoculation, and he ordered that any doctor caught performing the procedure be put to death. It was not a fortuitous decision. Thomas caught smallpox himself and died on June 2 by which time the camp had become a "veritable pest hole."[45] At Sorel the sick were housed in filthy barns with maggots feeding on their necrotic sores.[46] Worms an inch long crawled out of their ears. Congress sent Charles Carroll, Samuel Chase, and Benjamin Franklin to Sorel to sort out the disaster. The committee was not optimistic: "We are unable to express our apprehension of the distress our army must soon be reduced to from the want of provisions and the smallpox."[47]

One of the best descriptions of military inoculation for smallpox came during the Continental Army retreat from Quebec in soldier Daniel Kimball's diary. On March 26, 1776, he traded two quarts of rum for a wagon ride to a place five miles from his camp to "have the smallpox." He was inoculated and sent to a tent to recover. That night "I was so weak that if I had not set down I must in necessity have fel down." He was hardly able to sleep that night and when he got up "it turned as dark as Midnight Darkness." Kimball was able to sleep a bit the next day and on the twelfth day he broke out in pox. Two days later the fever lessened, and he was able to eat for the first time although the French Canadians he paid $3 a day to care for him offered only soup. Five days later, "My pock turned and I went out a doors." Another ten days and he was back with his unit on garrison duty.[48] A couple of parts of the description are worthy of note. First he had no preparation prior to and no treatment after the procedure. Second he was apparently not quarantined after the procedure, and he may well have still been contagious when he returned to his unit.

The remaining Continentals had withdrawn to a small island in the St. Lawrence where fifteen to twenty died of smallpox and were buried in shallow graves each day. By July those left were back at Fort Ticonderoga, but their suffering was not over.

TICONDEROGA

Maj. Gen. Horatio Gates, whom Washington had sent to take command at Ticonderoga, found a medical disaster. He wrote Washington on July 29, "Everything about this Army is infected with the Pestilence; the cloaths, the Blankets, the Air, & the Ground they walk upon."[49] Gates's first measure was to separate the infected from the healthy. He moved the smallpox quarantine hospital across the lake to Fort George, built a two-thousand-bed facility that was the largest hospital of the war, and staffed it with female camp followers as nurses.

At the fort anyone who got smallpox was required to take an oath that they had gotten it in "the natural way" so inoculators could be caught and punished. Gates suspected that men were getting inoculated so they would not have to fight and could still collect what he considered inordinately generous sick pay. Besides, his force was plagued by desertions, which he informed Washington were largely from fear of smallpox. Desertions threatened the civilian population as well; deserters took smallpox with them when they returned to Massachusetts, Connecticut, and New York.

But rigid quarantine and widespread self-inoculation worked. On August 28, Gates informed Washington that the epidemic in his Northern Army was over.

WASHINGTON AND INOCULATION

There was one more outbreak in 1776, but that one worked to Washington's advantage. Lord John Murray, the last royal governor of Virginia, promised freedom to the slaves of any revolutionaries who would agree to fight with

Loyalist forces. The exact number of slaves who accepted the offer is not certain, but somewhere between eight hundred and two thousand enlisted in the "Ethiopian Regiment." Murray had fled the Governor's Palace at Williamsburg and taken residence on HMS *Fowey* anchored at Yorktown. Early in 1776 smallpox broke out in his troops after they came ashore at Tucker's Point near Portsmouth, and the outbreak spread among the refugee slaves. The Loyalists abandoned Tucker's Point for Gwynn's Island some fifty miles to the north, leaving three hundred dead buried in shallow graves. But smallpox went with them, and escaped slaves continued to drift in and get sick. Murray was convinced his Ethiopian Regiment would have grown to two thousand men save for the disease, but the regiment was down to a mere three hundred when he finally gave up and left Virginia on July 9, 1776.

General Sir Henry Clinton, who had assumed command of British forces in North America in February 1778, tried to enlist slaves as well. He issued the Phillipsburg Proclamation freeing all slaves owned by revolutionaries on June 30, 1779, and perhaps as many as 100,000 of them attempted to escape over the course of the war. Thomas Jefferson estimated that 30,000 from Virginia alone had joined the British, but that 27,000 of those had died either of smallpox or camp fever.[50]

By spring 1776 it was obvious that the risk of smallpox to the army in Boston and the disaster that befell the retreating army in New York must not be repeated. Even the seat of the Continental government in Philadelphia was a problem. Because quarantine regulations and licensing restrictions on inoculation had been sporadically enforced, the city was a hotbed of smallpox. Inoculations had been suspended while the Continental Congress met in 1774, but the practice resumed after a brief hiatus, and people came from around the colonies for the procedure. Patrick Henry was inoculated by Dr. Benjamin Rush; Washington insisted that his wife be inoculated if she were to continue to visit him in camp, and after objecting she came to Philadelphia for the procedure as well.[51]

Washington was gradually moving toward mandatory inoculation. In June 1776 he tried to convince the Virginia legislature to require the masters of each household to inoculate every newborn, both slave and free. That requirement did not, however, extend to his troops. Mass inoculation would take his army out of service for weeks. Besides, those inoculated would have to leave infected clothing behind, and Washington had nothing with which to replace it. In the summer of 1776, after having moved the bulk of his forces to New York, Washington ordered inoculations to stop and ordered that any local physicians caught inoculating be jailed. But Boston was a caution. In July Dr. James Warren wrote John Adams that the arrival in the city of copies of the Declaration of Independence was a great relief since all anyone had been talking about was smallpox, and the whole city had become one "great hospital for inoculation."[52]

Washington's inoculation ban was not working out well. It made recruiting to the Northern Army difficult since potential enlistees were unwilling to risk infection, and his generals were not enforcing it. The practice was resumed in upstate New York, and inoculation quarantine hospitals were set up in remote farms. Washington's fear of taking men out of service was borne out when Brig. Gen. Samuel Holden Parsons said the number of men under inoculation and those required to care for them made it impossible to send reinforcements to resist the British landing at Long Island in 1776.

Smallpox followed Washington in his retreat from New York. By the time the Continentals set up camp across the river from Trenton the Pennsylvania enlistments were about to expire. In a masterful display of leadership Washington convinced almost all of them to stay, but in a matter of weeks almost half were dead from either wounds or smallpox. Some 11,000 men fought in the December 26 Battle of Trenton; by early January 1777 only 1,400 remained.

The decision to inoculate or not was now entirely in the hands of a Virginia planter with limited education and command experience who had been out of the country only once and had only visited a city one time before the Revolution. Although he had enough mathematics to be a surveyor, he had no background in either medicine or science. Physicians and Congress could make recommendations, but Washington had absolute power, and he was in a quandary. William Shippen Jr., Director General of Hospitals West of the Hudson, wrote from Philadelphia, "The smallpox raises & it is the opinion of the committee of Congress & the generals that inoculation should take place immediately in such manner as that those who pass & repass hereafter (referring to transit through Philadelphia), may not be liable to receive infection unless circumstances may make it proper. It is 3 to 1 that all in town have taken the infection & will carry it to the Army unless inoculated."[53] But Shippen could only offer an opinion. The decision rested with Washington; only he could mandate inoculation.

In a letter to Gates on February 5–6 Washington wrote: "I am much at a loss what Step to take to prevent the spreading of the smallpox; should We inoculate generally, the Enemy, knowing it, will certainly take Advantage of our Situation; 'Till some good Mode can be adopted, I know of no better than to alter the Route of the Troops marching from the South; You will therefore command all such to pass by way of Newtown, and not to touch at Philad under the most certain and severe Penalty."[54] Perhaps he could avoid spreading smallpox by keeping his recruits away from concentrations of civilians, but he knew that would not be enough.

As we have seen Washington was no stranger to smallpox. He had the disease himself and struggled to convince his wife to be inoculated. His army had been threatened by the virus in Boston, and he was convinced the British had tried to use it as a weapon. He had lost an army in Canada and, had Gates not quarantined and inoculated the Northern Army, the Revolution might well have been lost.

His New England recruits did not need to be convinced to be inoculated, but the same was not true of his rural southerners. Besides, inoculation would take his army out of service for several weeks. It was not an easy decision.

After a night's contemplation, Washington wrote Shippen, "Finding the smallpox to be spreading much and fearing that no precaution can prevent it from running through the whole of our Army, I have determined that the troops shall be inoculated. . . . Necessity not only authorizes but seems to require the measure, for should the disorder infect the Army in the natural way and rage with its usual virulence we should have more to dread from it than from the Sword of the Enemy."[55]

The general inoculation of Washington's troops was to be done in secret so the British would not know how many men were incapacitated, and Shippen was to do the same with all troops in Philadelphia. "I would fain hope they will be soon fit for duty, and that in a short space of time we shall have an Army not subject to this greatest of all calamities that can befall it."[56] Washington wrote President of the Continental Congress John Hancock informing him of the decision and reassuring him that recruits would lose no real time since they could recover while their "clothing and accoutrements" were being readied.[57] He asked for neither authorization nor support. The decision was his and it was made. For the next year, the Continental Army provided free inoculation and required it.

A week after the fact the Medical Committee of the Continental Congress wrote Washington to "consult him on the propriety and expediency of causing such of the troops in his army, as have not had the smallpox, to be inoculated, and recommend that measure to him, if it can be done consistent with the public safety, and good of the service."[58] The committee left the responsibility solidly with the general who had already made the decision.

Washington established inoculation hospitals in communities around Morristown so both his non-immune troops and the civilians in contact with them could be immunized. One hospital in the Moravian settlement at Bethlehem spread smallpox from troops to the town, and only inoculation of the entire civilian population averted an epidemic.

In April Dr. John Morgan recommended universal inoculation with the Dimsdale method, and inoculation hospitals were established in cities along the route southern recruits took on their way to join the army. The largest was at Alexandria with others at Dumfries and Colchester. Hundreds of North Carolina troops passed through the Alexandria facility, but it was not all smooth. Dr. William Rickman, deputy director general of the Southern Department, was fired when Virginia and Carolina recruits reported that their fellows were dying in the hospital after inoculation. Nicholas Creswell, passing through Alexandria, visited the hospital: "Such a pock-eyed place I was never in before."[59] A subsequent investigation found that the deaths were actually due to fatigue, poor clothing, and camp diseases other than smallpox, and Rickman was reinstated.[60]

By spring inoculation of all recruits was standard procedure, and the numbers were clear testimony to the wisdom of Washington's decision; mortality from "natural" smallpox hovered at around 16 percent while that from inoculation dropped to only 0.33 percent, and the army was largely free of the disease. Mandatory free inoculation had also removed a significant social divide—immunity was no longer confined to those with the money to pay for it.

Smallpox was key to the turning point of the Revolution. The Battle of Saratoga in September and October 1777 was radically different from the upstate New York experience a year earlier. Officers were expected to have healthy troops, sick soldiers were rigorously isolated, and the army was inoculated. A healthy army under Gates and Arnold defeated Burgoyne at Saratoga.

The British recognized that the center of enthusiasm for independence was in New England and reasoned that, if those colonies were cut off from the Middle and Southern colonies, the uprising would fail. In February 1777 British General John Burgoyne proposed leading troops from Canada down the Lake Champlain–Hudson Valley corridor to meet a force under General William Howe that would move up the Hudson from New York City, while a secondary force of British troops and allied Native Americans all under Lieutenant Colonel (Brevet Brigadier General) Barry St. Leger would strike east along the Mohawk River from Lake Ontario. The three armies would come together in upstate New York. Burgoyne took Fort Ticonderoga, and the plan looked to succeed until Howe went south to attack Philadelphia rather than going north to meet Burgoyne. St. Leger was stymied at Fort Stanwix and withdrew. Following the two battles of Saratoga (September 19 and October 7) Burgoyne, left alone and defeated, was forced to surrender to Gates.

Saratoga was a decisive victory. Perhaps most importantly, the battle helped convince the French government to come into the war on the Patriot side. Had the Continental Army not brought a smallpox epidemic under control this decisive victory would not have been possible, and the British might well have won the war.

When his army went into winter quarters at Valley Forge in 1777, Washington decided to continue the mass inoculation after closing the way station inoculation hospitals and moving the entire process to his headquarters. New men marched around the cities and were kept as fresh and healthy as possible on the march to prepare them for inoculation. Washington hoped less fatigued men would recover more quickly, an important consideration since his army—which had numbered 14,122 in December 1777—was down to 7,316 by March. He could ill afford to have recruits spending two or three weeks in Alexandria. Washington got word that Clinton was preparing to move his troops from Philadelphia to New York, and he wanted to attack them as they crossed New Jersey, but he would have had to leave 3,800 of his men behind since they were either recently inoculated or were caring for those who had been. Washington had to wait, but he was lucky. When Clinton actually moved in June the number in the hospital had dropped to around nine hundred, and those were being cared for by women newly enlisted as nurses rather than by their fellow soldiers. Washington's army was back at strength.

By 1778 the army was essentially free of smallpox, and mandatory inoculations were suspended. Smallpox remained a sporadic problem for the Continental Army through 1782, but it never posed the same threat as in 1775. In January 1781 there were cases in Maj. Gen. Nathanael Greene's North Carolina troops, possibly contracted from prisoners of war although there was also an outbreak among local civilians. Greene, unwilling to take his men out of service long enough to be inoculated, banned the procedure, but the outbreak died out on its own.

In June 1781, Connecticut soldier Josiah Atkins claimed that British Major General Lord Charles Cornwallis had inoculated some four to five hundred former slaves and sent them into American lines. The following month Major General Alexander Leslie wrote Cornwallis that he intended to scatter seven hundred inoculated refugee slaves among rebel plantations. Whether either of these actions was actually taken is uncertain, but by that time most of the Continental Army and its camp followers were immune. In January 1782, the disease briefly resurfaced in Washington's Northern Army, and he instituted a new campaign to inoculate every non-immune soldier. That month two thousand men were inoculated; the project was complete by May, and the outbreak was controlled.[61]

In the COVID-19 epidemic vaccine mandates created seismic political rifts. Between December 14, 2020, and December 20, 2021, 496 million vaccine doses were administered with 10,688 deaths reported after those inoculations. Every death following vaccination was reported regardless of whether that death was the result of vaccination or simply coincident, and even if every death had been caused by the vaccine the mortality rate was only 0.004 percent for a two-dose course; had the death rate from COVID-19 vaccination been the same as for smallpox inoculation in the eighteenth century, 10 million might have died. From that perspective Washington's decision to inoculate his army was remarkable—and remarkably effective.

In 1776 there was no legislative, judicial, or executive mechanism for mandating inoculation of the Continental Army. Washington, with no official authorization, ordered inoculation of his entire army. Inoculation rendered the soldiers ineffective for weeks. It made them a danger to uninoculated civilians. It carried an anticipated 2 percent mortality. And it worked. Of the four tools for combatting an epidemic, mandated immunization may be the best suited to a military force, and it may have saved the Revolution.

CHAPTER 2

ECOLOGY

Typhoid in Two Wars

While war and famine, inundations and earthquakes destroy
their thousands, febrile miasms bring millions to the grave. . . .
Even when death does not occur, the effects of fever are
often more painful and grievous than those of mortal hurts,
or from mechanical violence.

—*Transylvania Journal of Medicine and Associate Science*
(November 1830)

Soldiers have rarely won wars. They more often mop up after
the barrage of epidemics. . . . The epidemics get the blame
for defeat, the generals the credit for victory.

—Hans Zinsser, *Rats, Lice and History*
(1934)

THE RECORD

Although an unprecedented volume of medical data was compiled during and after the Civil War, it is difficult to accurately assess the impact of specific infectious diseases between 1861 and 1865. While the war was still going on Congress authorized the Office of the Surgeon General of the Army to collect data on injuries and illnesses suffered by Union soldiers resulting in the six-volume *Medical and Surgical History of the War of the Rebellion* that tips in at a shelf-straining sixty pounds. Three of the volumes are essentially tables and graphs of the diseases—mostly infections—that plagued the Union armies. Swiss-German microbiologist Theodor Edwin Klebs said the massive undertaking left "anything that ever since has been achieved in Europe way in the background."[1]

The amount of data is breathtaking, but it suffers from two serious shortcomings. First it is a compilation of the Union experience. There is no similar set of data for the Confederate forces, and that problem is compounded by the fact that the largest store of data from the Southern states was lost in a Richmond warehouse fire near the war's end. What was left is mostly records kept by individual military surgeons and some hospitals, and it is difficult to compare to the Northern experience.

The second problem is more a matter of medicine than of data. Coming before general acceptance of the germ theory, the Civil War was the last major conflict in which diseases were classified based on their symptoms rather than their causes. Except for a few exanthemata like measles and smallpox, infections were sorted according to the pattern of fever associated with them, and those diagnoses were inexact and regularly incorrect.

Inaccurate diagnosis was complicated by the fact that there was almost never a time in which disease did not materially affect the conduct of campaigns, especially early in the war.[2] Measles, mumps, and diphtheria plagued recruits in the first years. Diarrhea and dysentery including typhoid, paratyphoid, and cholera accompanied every campaign and were particularly severe in both Union and Confederate prisoner-of-war camps. Seasonal respiratory disease was rampant throughout. Nonetheless, official reports by line officers, postwar memoirs, and many recent in-depth histories of the war hardly mention disease at all. Former Confederate Lt. Gen. James Longstreet's monumental memoir devotes almost one hundred pages to an hour-by-hour description of the Peninsular Campaign without a single mention of the typhoid and dysentery that plagued both sides.[3] Gen. Robert E. Lee's memoirs are the same as many recent multivolume histories of the war. To get a firsthand picture of the impact of epidemics on the war it is necessary to go to the letters and diaries of the participants where descriptions of disease and the incident suffering are plentiful.

We will start with an overall picture of the state of American military medicine and the incidence and (as far as possible) the types of infections that plagued the soldiers and how they were dealt with. Then we will look at one pivotal campaign where disease was key to the outcome.

THE MEDICAL BUREAU

The Union Army started the war with some 15,000 men scattered in small commands led by superannuated officers many of whom were relics of the Mexican War, and it ballooned to almost 500,000 cursorily screened men most of whom had little experience with or immunity to epidemic diseases. Army physicians "examined" up to ninety recruits an hour. The fact that four hundred women were enlisted as men is indicative of the thoroughness of those exams.[4]

When the war started the Medical Bureau was commanded by Surgeon General Thomas Lawson, who had been in the Army for fifty-five years and had accompanied Gen. Winfield Scott on the march from Vera Cruz to Mexico City in 1847. On May 15, 1861, Lawson had a fatal stroke and was succeeded by Clement Finley who was a mere eight years younger. Finley had served in the Black Hawk War (1832), the Seminole War (1838), and with Gen. Zachary Taylor in the Mexican War (1846–48).

Frederick Law Olmstead, whom we will meet later, thought Finley vain and incompetent, and he vigorously and unsuccessfully opposed the appointment. Olmstead's personal animosity aside, Finley was completely unequipped to manage the bureau's explosive growth. He took great pride in his parsimony and regularly spent less on drugs and medical supplies than Congress allocated. Finley preferred to wait until after a battle was fought to decide what he needed, assuming he could find surgeons and supplies from civilian sources if they were really necessary. The entire Medical Bureau administration comprised only three clerks and a handful of stewards. The bureau had no hospitals, no nurses, and only a few miserably uncomfortable ambulances. Resignations and dismissals for disloyalty at the beginning of the war cut the Army's 114 surgeons to 98. Finley officially retired April 15, 1862, and the bureau was reorganized, but for the first year of the war medical care in the Union Army was dismal.

The Confederate Medical Corps, although poorly equipped, was at least less chaotic. Three surgeons and twenty-nine assistant surgeons who resigned from the Union Army were the heart of a service modeled after that of the service they had left. In February 1861, the Confederate Congress authorized a surgeon general, thirty surgeons, and eighty-three assistant surgeons along with one surgeon and one assistant surgeon to be contracted for each regiment and $50,000 to construct military hospitals. President Jefferson Davis named Charleston physician Samuel Preston Moore surgeon general on July 30, 1861, just after the Battle of Manassas (First Battle of Bull Run). Moore would serve through the entire war as the Confederate Medical Corps grew to some 3,500 officers.

After 1862, the Union Medical Bureau ballooned as well. Congress authorized ten surgeons and twenty assistant surgeons for the regular department who primarily served in administrative positions. General hospitals were staffed by 107 brigade surgeons and 5,532 "acting assistant surgeons" serving without commissions. Most remained under contract, although some were only waiting to sit exams that would allow them to become officers. Each volunteer state regiment brought its own surgeon, most of whom were chosen more for their connections than their clinical ability. By the end of the war 12,343 physicians had served in the Medical Bureau (about six for every hundred men), although almost none came with experience treating either battle injuries or epidemics.[5]

After the Battle of Bull Run wounded Union soldiers had been left lying in the field for as long as three days because there were not enough ambulances to transport them or hospitals to treat them. Newspaper reports of their suffering were a national scandal aggravated by the fact that the camps around Washington, D.C., were rife with epidemic disease, and government officials were acutely aware of the possibility that disease could spread from the soldiers to civilians including themselves.

REFORM

A chance encounter on a New York City sidewalk between the Reverend Doctor Henry Whitney Bellows, pastor of All Souls Unitarian Church, and prominent local physician Dr. Elisha Harris initiated a solution. Both were aware of the disaster that befell British troops in the Crimean War as a result of poor sanitation and abysmal medical care, and they were determined that the experience not be repeated in the War of the Rebellion. They joined a group of concerned women at Cooper Union to form the Women's

Central Association of Relief with a group of officers all of whom were, ironically, men. The group's first initiative was a nursing course for women at Bellevue Hospital, but the long-term goal was to start a sanitary commission modeled after that formed in Britain in response to the Crimean failure. The group joined two other voluntary relief societies and renamed itself the United States Sanitary Commission before offering its services to the Medical Bureau. Senior officers in the bureau tersely informed them that the department was "fully competent" to meet the war's demands. Their help and interference were unnecessary.

A delegation of the disappointed volunteers traveled to Washington to meet with Surgeon General Lawson. He was sick at home—not an unusual state of affairs—so they met with his assistant Dr. R. C. Wood, who was entirely aware of the department's shortcomings. Wood asked Secretary of War Simon Cameron to appoint a commission composed of a medical officer and five civilians—two of whom were to come from the New York delegation—to investigate sanitary conditions in the Army. Wood anticipated uncontroversial recommendations like better examination of recruits, better training for cooks, use of newly trained female nurses, and hiring medical students to change dressings and help on the wards. President Abraham Lincoln was skeptical of even modest changes, referring to the commission as "the fifth wheel on a coach."[6] After he replaced Lawson, Finley reluctantly accepted the commission provided they only investigate and advise and agree not to meddle with regular troops. Lincoln signed the order creating the commission on June 13, but he and Finley got a great deal more than they bargained for.

The commission chose Frederick Law Olmstead executive secretary and set to work. When Lawson died the New York group had lobbied to have Wood replace him, but Lincoln, bowing to seniority, appointed Finley instead. Olmstead and the commission embarked on a crusade to get rid of the "old codger" and to reform the entire Medical Bureau in the process. First they appointed six distinguished physicians to examine the camps around Washington. Given the realistic civilian concern about the spread of infections from the camps to the community and the sorry condition of supply and housing in the camps, it was a mission guaranteed to be popular with the public. Of the camps examined the commission found 5 percent "admirable," 45 percent "fairly clean," 26 percent "negligent," and 24 percent "decidedly bad, filthy, and dangerous."[7] The *Tribune* declared the bureau "simply inefficient and inert," and the editors castigated its officers for spending more time fighting with the commission than with "its natural and official enemies" typhus, malaria, and smallpox. But the bureau had its supporters. The *New York Times* accused the commission of "meddling mischievously with matters which are already in competent and experienced hands" and said it was "bitten by the ambition of superseding (sic), or at least remodeling, the established Medical Bureau of the regular army."[8] In the last they were quite right.

The commission won. On April 16, 1862, Congress passed a bill to reorganize the bureau. The surgeon general's rank was increased to brigadier general, the staff was expanded, and eight "medical inspectors" with rank between the surgeons and the surgeon general were appointed. The commission recommended a long list of medical supplies to be purchased, but new Secretary of War Edwin Stanton agreed with regular army surgeons that the list was bloated and reflected the whims of volunteer surgeons who knew nothing of actual military needs. The commission was forced to appeal to the general public for wine, spirits, ice, bedding, and mosquito nets.

The recalcitrant Medical Bureau was, however, about to undergo a dramatic change. Finley was ousted, and his replacement was a different man altogether. William Hammond was born in Annapolis, raised in Harrisburg, and graduated from the Medical Department of the University of the City of New York. He spent time at the Pennsylvania Hospital where he studied under Silas Weir Mitchell, the father of American neurology. Hammond joined the Army in 1849, and he spent the next decade moving from one small western post to another before Mitchell talked him into leaving the Army for academic medicine. With epic poor timing Hammond resigned his commission early in 1860. When the war started he rejoined the Medical Bureau, but he was dropped to the bottom of a seniority list that determined rank and promotion.

Despite his lack of seniority the Sanitary Commission knew Hammond's exemplary record as Brig. Gen. William Rosecrans' medical officer, and they lobbied Stanton and Lincoln to have him replace Finley. The

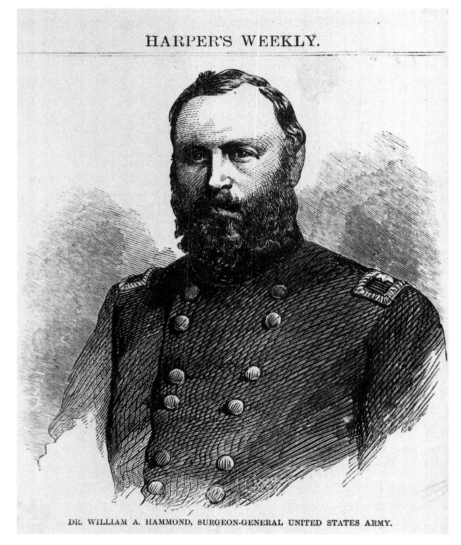

HARPER'S WEEKLY.

DR. WILLIAM A. HAMMOND, SURGEON-GENERAL UNITED STATES ARMY.

Surgeon General William A. Hammond introduced fundamental reforms to the Union Medical Bureau. *National Library of Medicine*

Sanitary Commission saw Hammond as a man with military experience who was not part of the ossified hierarchy that had proven so incompetent. To the unremitting distress of most army surgeons, Hammond was promoted directly from lieutenant to surgeon general over almost the entirety of the Medical Corps.

Hammond was arrogant, opinionated, and generally impossible to get along with. One of his associates said he was "rarely anything but captious, irritable, and pompous."[9] The new surgeon general met with Stanton two days after his appointment, and at the height of a heated discussion informed the secretary that, "I am not accustomed to be spoken to in that manner by any person. . . . I will not permit you to speak to me in such language as you have just used." Stanton replied, "Then, sir, you can leave my office immediately."[10] The relationship only got worse, but Hammond managed to accomplish a great deal before things fell apart completely.

He appointed Jonathan Letterman medical inspector general, and the evacuation system for the wounded was radically redesigned. He recruited a hospital corps that grew to eleven men for every one hundred patients. He put the corpsmen in uniform, subjected them to military discipline, and paid them $20.50 a month when nurses were receiving only $0.50 a day. In fiscal 1862, the bureau had not even spent all of its $2,445,000 budget. In 1863 Hammond spent $11,594,000, a full $1,250,000 more than was allocated that year.

Hammond also removed calomel and tartar emetic from the Army supply list. The mercurials were the two most popular drugs in the formulary, and they were seen as panaceas by military surgeons, especially those attached to volunteer regiments. Hammond correctly believed they rarely did any good and were frequently harmful, but his doctors disagreed and took the argument to the secretary of war.

The conflict between the surgeon general and his boss was exacerbated by the conflict over the appointment of the medical inspectors who occupied a position between surgeons and the administration in Washington. Hammond expected they would be chosen based on experience and clinical expertise. Stanton and members of Congress saw the positions as political favors and chose appointees that included Inspector General Thomas Perley who was said to be distinguished primarily for his imbecility. Hammond was livid.

In July 1863, Stanton took advantage of the uproar over calomel and tartar emetic and appointed a special commission chaired by Andrew J. Reeder, one of Hammond's sharpest critics, to examine the surgeon general's papers and records. J. K. Barnes was made interim surgeon general, and Hammond was court-martialed and dismissed from the Army on August 30, 1864.

He returned to New York where he achieved considerable success with his expertise in neurology. In 1878, the verdict was reversed, and Hammond was promoted brigadier general and awarded back pay for the time since his court-martial. He accepted the commission, but he refused the back pay. The Sanitary Commission gave Hammond the lion's share of the credit for reforming the Medical Bureau and for the dramatic improvement in medical care in the Union Army after 1862.

INFECTION IN THE FIRST MONTHS

Meanwhile, there had been the winter of 1861–62 when both the North and the South had seen infectious disease run rampant. Measles, diarrhea, dysentery, and typhoid were all epidemic, and 20–50 percent of the men in every unit in the east were sick. Sanitation was ignored, latrines were filthy and mostly unused, and clouds of flies swarmed every camp. The "hospitals" were mostly regimental infirmaries staffed by inexperienced and incompetent surgeons. The only nurses were soldiers, most of whom were men their commanding officers wanted to be rid of.

Maj. Charles Tripler was appointed chief surgeon of the Army of the Potomac in August 1861 and set out to reorganize the dysfunctional system. Regimental hospitals were abolished and replaced with a hierarchy of division, corps, and general hospitals. Tripler was described by a colleague as an energetic, spasmodic, crotchety, genial soul. He had been in the Medical Department since 1830 and was military through and through.

Tripler distrusted the general hospitals almost as much as the regimental ones. The early general hospitals were set up in hotels, schools, warehouses, and jails—wherever there was a roof and open space. Beds, bedding, dressings, and medicines were notably lacking. Most of the general hospitals were staffed by contract surgeons of widely variable training and ability. In Tripler's mind the worst part of the general hospitals was the tendency of contract surgeons to discharge recovered patients home rather than sending them back to their regiments.

Despite his distrust of hospitals, Tripler told the Bureau he would need 20,000 beds to meet the coming need. He seriously underestimated. By the end of 1862 there were over 90,000 sick and wounded in 151 Union general hospitals with 58,715 beds even though the majority of the sick were still being treated in field hospitals or had been discharged home.[11] By 1864 there were 204 general hospitals with 136,894 beds.[12] By the end of 1866 every one of those had closed.

The Confederacy had some 150 hospitals, mostly clustered around Richmond. The largest of these was in the heights above the James River and grew to 8,000 beds in 150 pavilions. Because five railroads converged on Richmond and much of the war was fought in Northern Virginia, Chimborazo was the largest hospital in the Confederacy by far, although it served mostly for recovery rather than acute treatment of trauma and saw far more disease than injury. Nursing was done by a few matrons, injured and recuperating soldiers, and slaves, and, although the facility was under-supplied, it was generally well organized. James B. McCaw, whose son Walter later served as the chief surgeon of the American Expeditionary Forces in World War I, was the hospital's only commander.

The Union general hospitals were decidedly unpleasant places. Because it was generally thought that moisture precipitated gangrene, the floors, rather than being washed, were "dry scrubbed" with sand. Foul bedding and used dressings littered the wards. Hospitals that had indoor toilets often did not have the water pressure to flush them, and many lacked running water altogether. Hammond described a hospital he visited in Cumberland, Maryland: "The condition of this building defies description. It is simply disgusting. The outhouses are filled with dirty clothes, such as sheets, bed sacks, shirts, & c., which have been soiled by discharges from sick men. The privy is fifty yards from the house, and is filthy and offensive ad nauseam. It consists of a shed built over two trenches. No seats; simply a pole, passing along each trench, for the men to sit on."[13]

Early in the war, enlisted men were admitted to hospital without charge; officers, on the other hand, had to pay $1.00 a day—with an additional $.30 if they had a personal servant—for the privilege of being hospitalized.

Surgeons, although they had no authority over regular military personnel, were in charge of patients and staff. The patients who were able were expected to stand at attention at their bedside when the surgeons made rounds, and at least one doctor insisted on being accompanied by a fife and drum as he strolled through the wards.[14] The level of medical care was generally on par with the surroundings.

MEDICINE IN 1861

Unfortunately the germ theory of infectious disease, although almost proven, was a decade away from general acceptance. In 1847, Ignaz Semmelweis figured out that bare-handed medical students going directly from the dissecting room to the delivery room were the cause of often fatal puerperal fever, but he did not publish his findings until 1860, and general acceptance of contamination as a cause of infection only came a couple of decades after that. In 1866, Louis Pasteur proved that bacteria caused wine to go bad, but his finding was not extended to human disease for another decade.

Absent an understanding of the cause, diseases were classified according to the pattern of fevers sorted into a mind-boggling array of categories. By 1860, fevers were usually divided into the following groups: intermittents that came and went on schedule, typically malaria; remittents that came, resolved, and then came back, mostly typhoid; and continuous fevers that came and stayed, most commonly sepsis or pneumonia. Those associated with skin rashes like smallpox or measles were lumped together as exanthemata and were joined by a bewildering and generally unhelpful array of classifications such as enteric fever, nervous fever, gastric fever, and intestinal bilious fever. The confusion surrounding fevers was made worse by the fact that Civil War physicians rarely measured a patient's temperature at all. Besides, except for malaria which was most often misdiagnosed, what the fevers were called was of virtually no therapeutic use.

Fevers were to be expected. In retrospective remarks to the International Medical Congress after the war, Army assistant surgeon and microscopist Joseph Janvier Woodward said,

> Since the earliest times Pestilence had followed the footsteps of war.
> It has been the consequence as much of Ignorance as of Necessity. Its
> causes are to be sought not merely in fatigues, exposures, and priva-
> tions necessarily incurred during the performance of heroic deeds;

not merely in the morbific influences of strange climates; not merely in the miseries of besieged places; they are equally to be sought in the thousand preventable abnormal conditions to which armies are exposed when huddled together in ill-selected, overcrowded, and filthy camps, fed by ignorance or cupidity in scanty, improper, ill-cooked food, drinking water contaminated by human excretions, and breathing air poisoned by human effluvia.[15]

During the war Woodward was sure the majority of camp diseases were caused by a combination of three factors: climate, mode of life, and diet. Climate caused intermittent fevers (malaria), mode of life—poor sanitation, exposure—caused typhus and typhoid, and inadequate diet caused scurvy. Woodward thought camp fevers resulted from a combination of the three and should be lumped into what he called typho-malarial fever with or without "scorbutic influences."[16] Unfortunately, the resulting confused and incorrect diagnoses hampers the usefulness of the *Medical and Surgical History* that Woodward coauthored. On the positive side, there was an emphasis on sanitation and control of mode of life risks. "Crowd poisoning," thought to come from air contaminated by emanations given off during respiration, led to larger wards and open windows. Removing "effluvia" from the skin led to cleaner bodies and cleaner clothes. Avoiding the decomposition of various normal and abnormal excreta lessened fecal contamination. The belief in "miasms" emanating from rotting organic matter in swamps and marshes discouraged camping in mosquito-ridden areas even though the insect's role in disease would not be clear for nearly another half century.

It was obvious that some diseases were contagious; there was no doubt that syphilis and smallpox passed from person to person, but gangrene was incorrectly included among the contagions, so patients with rotting limbs were quarantined in separate wards.

Many physicians still believed contagion rarely caused disease. Besides, quarantine was viewed as an infringement on personal liberty, and the anti-contagionists remained dominant until the last half of the nineteenth century when specific bacteria were incontrovertibly linked to a variety of diseases.

Most medicines were even less useful than sanitation or quarantine. Except for opiates for pain (or occasionally diarrhea), quinine for malaria, and chloroform and ether as anesthetics, the Civil War pharmacopeia was as useless as it was extensive. Purgatives, diuretics, and diaphoretics were used to wring presumed poisons out of the body. Mercury-containing drugs like calomel were used to promote salivation for the same reason, even though they had a distressing tendency to cause gum disease, jaw necrosis, and occasional renal failure and death. Mercurials were the most commonly used drugs in the Union formulary before Hammond tried to remove them. He stopped supplying calomel, but mercurials stayed around in other forms. It was rare for a Union surgeon to be without a mercury-containing wad of "blue mass" in his pocket from which a lump could be cut and administered for diarrhea or dysentery. The ubiquitous "blue pills" compounded out of mercury, licorice, rose petals, sugar, and honey served the same purpose.

Various quinine-containing concoctions were unquestionably useful in both preventing and treating malaria, and during the war the Medical Bureau dispensed nineteen tons of quinine and nine and a half tons of raw cinchona bark. Most often the quinine was mixed with whiskey so the men would take it. Unfortunately, quinine was also used for a variety of non-malarial fevers for which it was entirely useless, and it was regularly prescribed for pain relief as well.

Opiates were effective at controlling diarrhea although they did nothing about the underlying cause, but they were less aggressive than cauterizing the rectal mucosa with silver nitrate to scar the anal opening and slow diarrheal discharge.[17] Opiates were, however, effective pain relievers, and 3 million ounces were dispensed by Union surgeons.[18]

The Confederates were not so well supplied. The Union blockade effectively shut off the South's access to opiates and quinine, and Confederate surgeons were forced to fall back on an assortment of leaves and barks that were generally useless. Perhaps that was not all bad; in a May 1860 speech to the Massachusetts Medical Society, Oliver Wendell Holmes caustically said, "if the whole materiel medica, as now used, could sink to the bottom of the sea, it would be all the better for mankind,—and all the worse for the fishes."[19]

THE DISEASES

Despite the poor ability to diagnose, the paucity of useful treatments, and the abysmal hospital care, the surgeon general and his staff proclaimed themselves pleased with the bureau's performance in handling febrile diseases early in the war. To be fair Union medical statistics compared favorably both to prior American wars and to the European experience. The death rate from disease among American troops in the first year of the Mexican War was 110/1,000 men. In the Crimea that rate had been 341/1,000 among the French, 263/1,000 Russians, and 232/1,000 British troops.[20] In the first year of the Civil War the death rate from disease in the Union Army was 50.4/1,000 while that from wounds was 17.2/1,000.[21] Even in peacetime the Army had lost twenty-four men of every one thousand from disease. One can understand why Woodward, in his 1864 report to the surgeon general, felt the bureau was doing reasonably well.[22] But Union soldiers were five times as likely to get sick as civilians, and sick soldiers were profoundly affecting military operations. The hospitalization rate for intestinal disease was twenty-nine times what it would be in World War I, and the death rate from gastrointestinal illness was 258 times as high.[23]

Epidemics in both Union and Confederate armies came in waves. The first arrived with the influx of new volunteers at the beginning of the war. Those volunteers were largely from rural communities, and many had not been exposed to the usual childhood infectious diseases. In the year ending June 30, 1862, the Union Army recorded 21,672 cases of measles, a number that grew to 676,763 among the white troops with a 6 percent mortality by the end of the war.[24] In July 1862 the Sanitary Commission told Lincoln that 25 percent of the volunteer army was so unhealthy it was "not only utterly useless, but a positive encumbrance and embarrassment."[25] The numbers tailed off toward the end of the war, but the influx of Black recruits in 1863–64 brought another wave. Among the 8,555 new Black troops the death rate from infection was a staggering 11 percent.[26]

Not surprisingly, the rate among the Confederates was even higher. Among 10,000 troops in the Southern Army of the Potomac (which became the Army of Northern Virginia) between July and September 1861 there were 4,000 measles cases.[27] Pneumonia, bronchitis, otitis, and diarrhea were all common sequelae of measles, and Confederate surgeon Bedford Brown wrote, "The diseases consequent to and traceable to measles cost the Confederate Army the lives of more men and greater amount of invalidation than all other causes combined."[28] Lee said, "All the conscripts we have received are thus affected so that instead of being an advantage to us, they are an element of weakness, a burden. I think, therefore, that it would be better that the conscripts be assembled in camps of instruction so that they may pass through these inevitable diseases."[29] The recommendation was not followed. In December 1861, Gen. Alfred Sidney Johnston said that only 54,004 of his 91,988 troops were on duty; 37,984 were absent sick through a combination of measles, pulmonary disease, and diarrhea.[30] One can only guess what Johnston or Brig. Gen. P. G. T. Beauregard would have done at Shiloh with so many additional troops.

Once the recruits were "seasoned" by acquiring immunity to childhood diseases, they were subject to the second wave of respiratory disease, smallpox, and erysipelas. When pneumonia, bronchitis, and influenza are lumped together, the Union Army suffered some 1,765,000 cases with about 45,000 deaths during the war.[31] As with measles Black Union troops were more likely to die from pulmonary disease than their white counterparts, but it was worse for the Confederates who had a death rate from bronchitis and pneumonia roughly five times that of Union troops.

Smallpox should not have been a problem since there was a proven vaccine, but a large percentage of volunteers on both sides were unvaccinated until Tripler made vaccination mandatory in October 1861. The smallpox rate is uncertain because it was often confused with chicken pox, but a rate of 5/1,000 troops is probably fairly accurate. As the war progressed vaccination itself became a problem because physicians were harvesting serum from vaccinated soldiers, in effect reusing vaccines. Some of the men also vaccinated themselves using pins, penknives, or any available sharp instrument without bothering to sterilize them. In addition to local infections, those vaccinations caused an undetermined number of cases of syphilis.[32] At the Battle of Chancellorsville in May 1863, five thousand of Lee's men were unable to report because they were sick from "spurious vaccination" presumed to be syphilis but possibly just other bacterial contaminants.[33] In all, the Union Army recorded 12,236 cases of smallpox with 4,717 deaths during the war.[34]

There was one smallpox case worth mentioning. Shortly after his Gettysburg speech Abraham Lincoln became the last American president to contract the disease. The press euphemistically termed the presidential illness "varioloid," but Lincoln spent November and December 1863 recovering. During his illness he remarked with regard to a waiting room full of petitioners, "There is one good thing about this. Now I have something I can give everybody."[35]

Early in the war the Confederates expected yellow fever to be their savior. Southerners were convinced that Yankees would die in droves during "fever season." For reasons that are not altogether clear yellow fever epidemics never materialized. There was a confined outbreak in Key West, and the disease broke out in the summer of 1862 on the USS *Delaware* at Hilton Head, South Carolina. It spread to local civilians three weeks later, but it never got beyond the island. Later in 1862 there were 1,507 cases in Wilmington, North Carolina, with a near 30 percent mortality, but again the disease remained local. There were, however, 21,691 cases of "jaundice" in the Union Army, and possibly, some of those were yellow fever. Confederates fully expected yellow fever to decimate the occupying Union Army in New Orleans, but that never happened, possibly because of Maj. Gen. Benjamin Butler's draconian sanitary regulations.

One of the war's more bizarre episodes involved Confederate surgeon Luke Pryor Blackburn's attempt to use yellow fever as a bioweapon. He went to Bermuda twice when the island was in the grip of an epidemic to collect clothing and bed linens from yellow fever patients. He shipped the contaminated items through Canada to the United States for resale. He even tried to send a fancy contaminated shirt as a gift to Lincoln, and Blackburn mistakenly believed that his infected clothing was responsible for the Wilmington outbreak. It would be one war later before physicians found out that it was mosquitoes, not dirty linens, that transmitted the disease.[36]

The real villains of the second wave of infections were dysentery, diarrhea, typhoid, and malaria. The diagnoses were muddled. Dysentery and diarrhea were symptoms of various bacterial or protozoal infections—enteropathogenic *Escherichia coli*, paratyphoid, cholera, *Shigella*, and *Giardia* along with *Entamoeba histolytica* that could lead to fatal chronic diarrhea. Diarrhea was diagnosed when frequent stools were not accompanied by tenesmus (the urge to defecate) while dysentery was, but it was a distinction without a difference. In the first half of 1861, 30 percent of the Union Army was sick, mostly with dysentery. In the year ending June 30, 1862, there were 212,449 cases of diarrhea reported, although there were likely as many more that never made the records.[37] In the entire course of the war there were 1,739,135 reported cases of diarrhea and dysentery with 44,558 deaths compared to 110,070 battle casualties.[38] By the end of the war, there had been 3,376 cases of diarrhea for every 1,000 troops—more than three cases per man.[39]

The Confederates were no better off. In Southern armies east of the Mississippi during the first two years of the war, there were 226,828 cases of diarrhea and dysentery reported in the field and an additional 86,506 in the hospital as compared to 29,569 gunshot wounds in the field and 47,724 in the hospital. In the same period battle wounds accounted for 4,241 deaths and dysentery 3,354.[40]

Disease, disability, and death caused by fecal contamination of food and water were preventable but predictable when hundreds of thousands of young men accustomed to having their clothes cleaned and their food prepared by their wives, mothers, and sisters moved away from home, crowded together, and were put on their own. Early in the war the Sanitary Commission published pamphlets intended to teach men to bathe and use latrines. When Jonathan Letterman became chief surgeon of the Army of the Potomac in June 1862, he ordered all meals to be prepared by company cooks rather than fried by individual soldiers. He had wells dug for fresh water, ordered tents to be aired out weekly, and tried to get the men to bathe once a week. Latrines were to be covered with six inches of fresh dirt every day and were separated from living spaces and camp kitchens. Kitchen offal and manure were to be buried. The situation got better as the war progressed, the men became more experienced, and sanitation improved.

As pervasive as dysentery was it affected both sides equally, and it rarely stopped military operations. The same was not true of malaria and typhoid. It is unfortunate that Woodward and his colleagues were so convinced that typhoid and malaria were one disease. That not only confused the record but also impacted treatment. Civil War surgeons were, of course, entirely unaware that malaria was caused by a mosquito-borne plasmodium and typhoid by fecal contamination with salmonella bacteria. One could be prevented by a drug and the other by sanitation, and the surgeons did not know the difference.

Both came with a fever, and that was all that counted. These "sthenic diseases" (as opposed to asthenic diseases like homesickness and depression) were characterized by congested blood vessels that evidently increased body heat, caused a fast pulse, and could culminate in delirium. Conventional treatment is aimed at drawing blood away from the center of febrile bodies, especially by "counterirritation." Bleeding had mostly been abandoned, but cupping, blistering the skin with mustard plasters, and turpentine wraps remained standard. Emetics and purgatives were thought to draw excess blood from the gastrointestinal tract, and leeches were applied to the abdomen and anus to achieve the same end. Diet was limited and protein intake was eliminated entirely to avoid "feeding the fever."[41]

Although they knew nothing of the actual cause, many Southern physicians had experience with malaria and knew the disease occurred in warm, low-lying, wet places. Outbreaks occurred after alluvial plains flooded and the water receded leaving fields of rotting vegetation, so, confusing correlation for causation, doctors concluded that rotting organic matter gave off disease-causing gases. A few observers did suggest that microscopic vegetable spores might be responsible, and Woodward allowed that idea might be worth further investigation at a later date.[42]

Fear of malaria did slow Union operations on the East Coast, especially in coastal South Carolina. Woodward considered the rice plantations around Charleston "extremely unhealthy," especially in the night air. If men had to be there he recommended they eat breakfast first thing so they would not go out before dawn, and he thought they should be restricted to their tents after dusk. His efforts to keep the troops out of the night air would keep them away from feeding mosquitoes, but he did not know that.

Dangerous areas could not always be avoided: "In many cases necessarily determined by pure military reasons, which cannot be overruled by any hygienic considerations, and the soldier, in the execution of his duty, must face diseases as he faces the bullets of the enemy—with patience and courage."[43] And they did. Between June 1861 and June 1862 there were 259 cases of intermittent fever for every 1,000 soldiers.[44] In the first year of the war, there were 77,096 cases of malaria reported in the 279,371-man Union Army.[45] Ultimately, there would be 1,028,750 cases (16 percent of reported illness) with 12,199 deaths among Union troops.[46] If anything the Confederates were worse off; they reported 164,726 cases of malaria with 2,182 deaths in the first year of the war alone.[47]

Perhaps the greatest military impact of malaria was at Vicksburg. The river town was one of the most malarious in the South with an incidence greater than Richmond, Memphis, Charleston, or New Orleans. The swamps behind the city were rife with the disease, and they protected the city from behind between May and July 1862 and forced Grant to attack from a different direction.

The positive with malaria was that, assuming the diagnosis was correct, it could be treated and even prevented. Whiskey mixed with quinine was used prophylactically in the Union Army beginning in 1861. The Sanitary Commission furnished the whiskey because the government would not, and the men took the drug primarily for the alcohol in which it was dissolved. The concoction was distributed only to men "fit for military duty" and was a powerful incentive for men to leave the hospital and return to their units.[48] Maj. Gen. Ulysses Grant's army in the west received five hundred barrels of bourbon in the spring of 1862. Although quinine had been used prophylactically by the Royal Navy since 1749 and had been used by the U.S. Army in Florida in 1840, its widespread use was one of the signal contributions of American military medicine during the Civil War.

The Confederates were, as usual, not so fortunate even though they were well aware of the value of quinine prophylaxis. The Union blockade essentially stopped quinine imports, so what supplies Southern physicians had were saved for the acutely ill. A variety of substitutes—tinctures of dogwood and poplar, willow bark dissolved in whiskey, and turpentine soaks—were tried with predictable futility.[49]

TYPHOID

Since both typhoid and malaria were fevers thought to be caused by miasms, it is likely that many if not most cases diagnosed as malaria or typho-malarial fever were actually typhoid. Diarrhea and dysentery may have been the most common diagnoses, but typhoid was the deadliest. *Salmonella typhi* is spread by the four Fs: fingers, flies, feces, and fomites. Humans are the only host for the organism, and the only way to get infected is from another person. Ingested bacteria adhere to and damage the intestinal lining, and lymphocytes and mononuclear cells attack the infected mucosa causing the pathognomonic ulcerations—Peyer's patches—that Civil War surgeons recognized as characteristic of typhoid, although their diagnostic usefulness was limited since the patches could only be seen at autopsy. Postmortem examinations were the result when the lesions ulcerated and perforated the intestine causing fatal peritonitis. Lesions that did not perforate could send bacteria into the bloodstream causing pneumonia, endocarditis, pancreatitis, osteomyelitis, aneurysms, and endotoxic shock. About 17 percent of patients got typhoid encephalopathy causing them to lay inert with half-open eyes awaiting coma and death.

Typhoid symptoms usually start twelve to forty-eight hours after exposure with nausea, vomiting, diarrhea, headaches, muscle aches, and anorexia. What Civil War surgeons knew as "continuous fever" increased in a stepladder fashion and could reach 105° Fahrenheit. Occasionally the fever would relent only to recur two or three weeks later. Stomach pain and a rose-colored skin rash were common signs. Diarrhea came with irritated bowel wall, although when the intestine became severely swollen it could obstruct the intestines and cause defecation to stop altogether.

Some 3–4 percent of survivors became asymptomatic carriers who could shed bacteria for years. Mortality from typhoid now is less than 1 percent, but in the Civil War it was fifteen to twenty times that. The disease remains common, affecting some 27 million people a year worldwide with about 215,000 deaths.[50] Wherever there is crowding, chaos, and poor sanitation the risk remains. For mid-nineteenth-century physicians it was almost impossible not to encounter the disease, and they were quite sure it came from airborne poisons. Woodward said, "The air is poisoned by putrid exhalations from the liquid discharges of diarrhea, dysentery, and

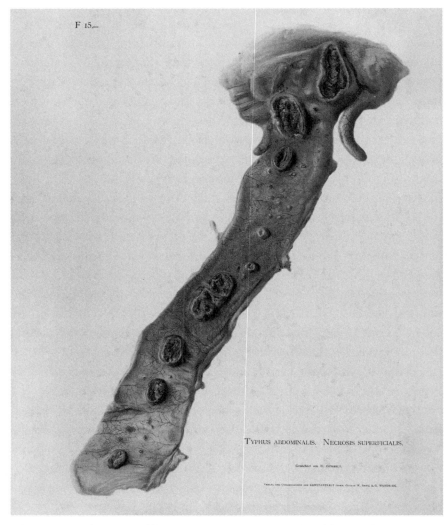

F 15.—

TYPHUS ABDOMINALIS. NECROSIS SUPERFICIALIS.

Ulcerations in the terminal ileum were typical in typhoid and frequently led to perforation of the bowel and fatal peritonitis. *Wellcome Library*

fever cases."[51] The Peyer's patches presumably gave off gases that allowed others to "inhale the very quintessence so to speak, of a pre-existing fever."[52] The anti-contagionists offered up an assortment of other possible causes of typhoid including sudden temperature changes, salted meat, stale vegetables, marsh miasms, impure emanations from close-packed bodies, and the lack of buoyancy and confidence.[53]

Military surgeons were all too familiar with "Tennessee trots," "Virginia quick step," alvine flux, and "Chickahominy fever," any of which might be E. coli, cholera, typhoid, or some other enteritis. During the war Union forces reported 75,418 cases diagnosed as typhoid among the white troops with a 36 percent mortality.[54] The incidence peaked between July 1862 and July 1863 when 5.9 percent of the Army was diagnosed with the disease and 2 percent of the entire force died from it. During 1861 and 1862 the Confederate Army reported 77,311 cases of "continuous fever" with 17,430 deaths.[55] As the war progressed and sanitation improved the incidence of typhoid declined, but the death rate increased from 17 percent to 56 percent, likely because the troops were more debilitated in the later years.[56]

So pervasive and lethal a disease had no shortage of suggested treatments. The diarrhea was treated with opiates, and Dover's powder—a combination of opium and ipecacuanha—remained in the formulary into the 1960s. Abdominal pain was treated with hot packs, blisters, and cupping. Fever was treated with cold packs to the head and cold-water sprays. Turpentine and arsenic were given by mouth in hopes of cauterizing intestinal ulcers. Brandy, ammonia, and capsicum were given for shock, and quinine was given since it worked for some fevers and might work for others. Oranges and lemon peel were administered to counter "scorbutic taint," another case of using one of the few things that worked. Vitamin C in citrus fruits cures scurvy but is of no use in typhoid.

Sanitary measures to control typhoid were not new in 1861. In 1854, English physician William Budd had written that typhoid was transmitted by infected feces and had proven it in a Munich epidemic in 1860. By 1863, the Sanitary Commission was pushing the "excreta theory" and arguing for disinfecting all privies with carbolic acid and chlorinated lime. In 1861, Tripler argued that the neglect of "plain hygienic principles" was responsible for most camp diseases.[57] The first three chapters of his manual for military surgeons dealt entirely with hygiene and dysentery. Gunshot wounds had to wait for later chapters. He gave detailed instructions for digging, maintaining, and disinfecting latrines and said, that although good hygiene might not eliminate dysentery, it would "so limit its prevalence as to make it no longer formidable."[58] But transmission by flies and asymptomatic carriers had yet to be demonstrated, and the anti-contagionists were quick to point out cases with no obvious fecal exposure.

THE WAR IN THE WEST

Tripler was right. Good hygiene might have shortened the war by two years, but before we get to the Peninsular Campaign, we need to take a short look at the war in the West. Johnston had withdrawn to Corinth where the Memphis to Charleston railroad spine of the Confederacy dipped into northern Mississippi after losing Forts Henry and Donelson to Grant. At the same time Johnston was joining Beauregard in Corinth, Maj. Gen. George McClellan was loading an armada of ships and barges with troops and materiel for an invasion of the Virginia peninsula bordered by the James and York Rivers.

Grant's and Johnston's armies came together April 6, 1862, at Shiloh chapel twenty-two miles northeast of Corinth. After two days in which more men were killed and wounded than in all previous American wars combined, the Confederates lost Johnston to a severed femoral artery and the battle to Grant's superior forces. Beauregard withdrew to Corinth.

Four days after the battle Maj. Gen. Henry Halleck arrived to assume command of the Union forces, and, after dragging out preparations for a month, marched into Corinth only to find that Beauregard had abandoned a town riddled with malaria and typhoid. Northern newspapers said the "victory" was tantamount to a defeat. The Confederates had left the area thoroughly contaminated, and Halleck's troops were almost immediately stricken with the "evacuation of Corinth" that left them too sick to pursue the retreating Southern army. Perhaps the signal effect of the occupation of Corinth was to instill Halleck with a fear of typhoid that dictated his decisions on the Virginia peninsula.

THE PENINSULA

Meanwhile in the East, McClellan had finally been pushed into the offensive against Richmond in which he would lose one-third of his army to dysentery, typhoid, and malaria. The expedition saw an average of three episodes of disease for every soldier during the next nine months.

McClellan's typhoid travails began that winter when he suffered a three-week bout of the disease himself. He had replaced superannuated Gen. Winfield Scott as general-in-chief of the Army November 1, 1861, and he had traveled to Hall's Hill, Virginia to review Maj. Gen. Fitz-John Porter's division three weeks later. Two days after that McClellan was too sick to report for work.

McClellan's support in Lincoln's cabinet had been shaky since Bull Run, and Attorney General Edward Bates took advantage of the general's absence to push Lincoln into taking a more active role in conducting the war. A Joint Committee on the Conduct of the War had been convened without McClellan, and it continued to meet after the general improved in January. McClellan's status was further hampered when the fever recurred midway through his recovery—not an uncommon event with typhoid.

When Lincoln tried to visit McClellan on January 8 he was told the general was too sick to receive visitors. The president then called Secretary of State William Seward, Secretary of the Treasury Salmon Chase, Assistant Secretary of War Thomas Scott, and Maj. Gens. Irvin McDowell and William Franklin, division commanders of the Army of the Potomac, to the White House to discuss attacking Richmond. McClellan was not invited. The committee's suggested options included another assault on Manassas Junction and an attack from the York River. McClellan, still suffering from typhoid, found out about the meeting four days later and was furious. He went to the White House, confronted Lincoln, and insisted on being invited to the committee's meeting the following day.

On January 13, Lincoln replaced Secretary of War Simon Cameron with Edwin Stanton to get "a stronger hand" to deal with McClellan. Lincoln and Stanton together pushed McClellan into what became the Peninsular Campaign. Although the general recovered from typhoid his influence was permanently eroded.[59] On January 27, Lincoln ordered the Army of the Potomac to attack at Manassas Junction by February 22, Washington's birthday. McClellan sent a twenty-two-page letter calling for an attack from Urbana on the Rappahannock River, but when Maj. Gen. Joseph Johnston moved his troops from the area around Washington to the south bank of that river the plan had to be changed.

McClellan convinced Lincoln that the next best route to Richmond was between the James and York Rivers up a seventy-five-mile long, fifteen-mile-wide peninsula from Fortress Monroe to the Confederate capital. On March 17, some 400 ships and barges left Annapolis with 50,000 men, a number that would grow to 121,500 before the campaign was over.

The advance up the peninsula started April 5. McClellan, a victim of inaccurate intelligence and excess caution, was convinced Johnston had 100,000 men dug in and waiting for him. Actually Brig. Gen. John B. Magruder had a scant 11,000 to delay the march until Johnston could bring his 43,000 men from Culpeper, Virginia. McClellan was beside himself when he learned that Lincoln had kept more than 50,000 men under Maj. Gens. Nathaniel Banks, John C. Fremont, and Irvin McDowell to chase Gen. Thomas "Stonewall" Jackson's army around the Shenandoah Valley and protect Washington.

The first battle of the campaign was fought May 5 at Fort Magruder where 41,000 Union troops clashed with 32,000 Confederates on the road between Yorktown and Williamsburg. After an inconclusive battle Johnston withdrew toward Richmond. Lincoln, Stanton, and Chase, who had come to witness a rout that never materialized, returned to Washington.

McClellan then made the near-fatal error of dividing his army into divisions on both sides of the Chickahominy River. The sluggish river arced east on the north side of Richmond before crossing the peninsula and emptying into the James River fifty miles to the south. Land on both sides of the Chickahominy was flat marsh that proved a formidable enemy for the Union.

Johnston took advantage of the divided Union army and attacked May 31. McClellan had 105,000 men to Johnston's 60,000 but was convinced he was outnumbered two to one. The Confederates suffered more casualties (6,134 to 5,031) and Johnston was severely wounded, but McClellan remained bogged down in the swamps and marshes along the Chickahominy.

Lee assumed command for the wounded Johnston and attacked on June 25. He managed to push McClellan as far as the plain at Malvern Hill where, on July 1, his army suffered severe casualties in an unsuccessful attempt to destroy the Union force. Despite the success at Malvern Hill,

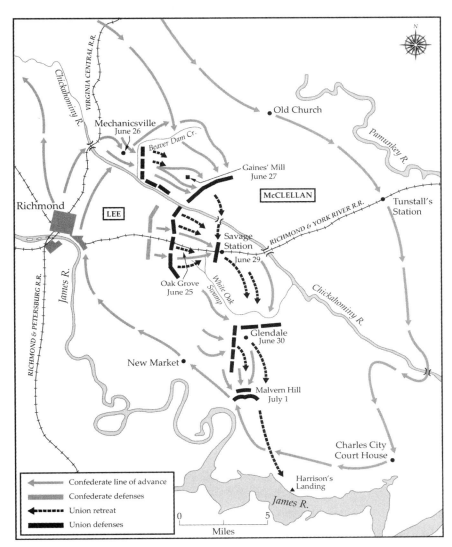

Map 3. The Peninsular Campaign

McClellan withdrew to Harrison's Landing on the James. Halleck, fresh from Corinth, insisted that what was left of McClellan's army get out of the swamp before fever season. For the time being Richmond was safe, and the Confederacy—at least in the East—looked to be winning. But the cost was high—15,849 Union casualties to 20,614 for the Confederates who could ill afford the loss.

When Johnston had withdrawn toward Richmond he took his men to higher, healthier ground, and left McClellan on poorly drained land contaminated with Confederate feces. In addition he was joined by Jackson's troops, almost all healthy after staying on the move through the Shenandoah Valley.

"Chickahominy Fever" was notorious among the Union troops. One New Hampshire surgeon wrote home, "The Chickahominy River . . . is a narrow, sluggish stream flowing through swamp land. This land is covered with a rank, dense growth of trees, reeds, grasses, and water plants. Vines climb and mosses festoon the trees; the soil is productive, but its stagnant water is poisonous; moccasins and malaria abound; flies and mosquitoes swarm; turtles and lizards bask; cranes and herons wade; buzzards and polecats slink; bitterns boo, owls hoot, foxes yelp, wildcats snarl and all nature seems in a glamor or a gloom."[60]

Johnston, responding to critics who wondered why he was not more aggressive, said, "I am fighting, sir, every day! Is it nothing that I compel the enemy to inhabit the swamps, like frogs, and lessen their strength every hour, without firing a shot?"[61]

After the Seven Days battle McClellan wrote Lincoln, "If, at this instant, I could dispose of 10,000 fresh men, I could gain victory tomorrow. I know that a few thousand more men would have changed this battle from a defeat to a victory. As it is, the government must not and cannot hold me responsible for the result."[62]

Lincoln never understood where all McClellan's men were. He reckoned that 160,000 men had been sent to the Peninsula by July 1862, and only 86,500 were left. Killed and wounded came to 28,500. Where were the other 45,000—more than four times what McClellan said would have won the campaign? They were sick.

Once off the Peninsula McClellan's army largely recovered, and although typhoid and malaria persisted through the remainder of the war sanitation improved. Union forces were out of the swamps, and diseases never again played as large a role in a military outcome as they did in 1862.

We need to take a brief look at the catastrophic death rate of prisoners of war on both sides. Union prisons saw some 6,000 deaths from dysentery,

5,000 more from respiratory disease, and about 3,500 from smallpox.[63] The Confederate prison at Danville, Virginia, had a 30 percent mortality from disease but that was eclipsed at Andersonville, the most notorious Confederate prisoner-of-war camp. The hospital there admitted 458 men for wounds or injuries and 15,987 for disease of whom 11,086 died.[64] Overall 15.5 percent of Union prisoners of war and 12 percent of Confederate prisoners died in the camps, virtually all from disease.[65] As tragic as those losses were, they did not affect the war's outcome since the men were already out of combat.

In sum the Civil War soldier was more at risk from disease than from combat. From April 15, 1861, to June 30, 1865, the average strength of the Union Army was 806,755 with a peak strength of 1,000,516. There were 110,070 battle-related deaths compared to 6,454,834 cases of reported illness with 224,580 deaths from disease.[66] Of all the deaths in the Civil War, 22.4 percent were from typhoid or "typho-malarial fever."[67]

The picture for the Confederates was grimmer. Manpower shortages forced the recruitment of older, less healthy men as the war progressed, and medical supplies and an increasingly effective Union blockade choked off the supply of drugs. The Confederates mobilized some 1,082,119 men with an average strength of 304,015. The Southern soldier on average suffered a disease or an injury six times during the war. In 1861–62, years for which there are some records, there were 797,290 men under treatment for fevers and dysentery as opposed to 77,293 being treated for wounds. Deaths from disease were 25,240 as opposed to 12,328 who either died in battle or later from wounds.[68] During the entire war, about 94,000 Confederate soldiers were killed in battle or died of wounds while about 164,000 died of disease.[69]

TYPHOID IN THE SPANISH-AMERICAN WAR

Typhoid in the early years of the Civil War should have been a well-learned lesson. It was not. What happened to the men who volunteered in 1898 repeated a monumental sanitation failure and accounted for the vast majority of the deaths in the war.

Of all the deaths in the Spanish war, 60.5 percent were from typhoid, and almost all were men who never left the United States.[70] One out of every five men who served in that war got the disease.[71] Just as in the prior war, typhoid arrived with inexperienced volunteers when they came together to learn soldiering.

The problem started in late April 1898 when more than 100,000 volunteers converged on state staging areas hastily thrown together with minimal planning and no attention to sanitation. The Army's few regular soldiers were accustomed to camp life, and many had learned hygiene the hard way in the Civil War. The new volunteers knew none of that, and their camps were uniformly filthy. One regimental surgeon said, "Look any time you would into the fields around that camp and you would see fifty to one hundred to two hundred men defecating."[72]

Like the state camps, the national cantonments in Virginia, Florida, Georgia, and Pennsylvania were thrown together with almost no attention to sanitation. Camp Thomas at Chickamauga Battlefield Park in Georgia was typical. When the camp ballooned to 60,000 men it poured out 9.4 tons of feces and 21,000 gallons of urine every day. It was built on thin soil over impermeable limestone, so the excreta pooled on the surface, and every pool was a potential typhoid reservoir.

By the time the regiments reported to the cantonments one-third of them already had typhoid, and that exploded to 98 percent within eight weeks.[73] When the short war ended the Army had lost the equivalent of twenty regiments to typhoid while only 243 men died in battle.[74]

When the men got typhoid their care was abysmal. Nursing was generally done by fellow soldiers who, without changing clothes or washing their hands, returned to their tents and mess halls at the end of the day to spread the disease. Conditions in the hospitals were awful. A *New York Times* reporter described one patient, "The man was ill of typhoid fever, and his temperature was above one hundred. When I reached his cot I nearly staggered with horror. The man's face was literally black with flies. His mouth, which was open—the poor fellow was too weak to close it—was filled with flies. . . . In another case a man who died in the division hospital was found to be literally alive with maggots beneath his armpits."[75]

Officers, especially junior ones, had no training in dealing with contagious diseases. The hygiene course at West Point mostly covered the adverse effects of alcohol, tobacco, and narcotics, and was taught by the

Department of Chemistry, Minerology, and Geology. Class notes were not required, and the course was not graded.

Army physicians, even if cognizant of basic hygiene, were only advisors to regular officers and had no authority over the camps or the men. Based on his experience in the Civil War, Surgeon General George Sternberg was quite certain that sanitation was essential, and within days of the declaration of war he issued Circular No. 1 with detailed instructions for keeping camps clean. The circular was ignored.

By the mid-1880s it had been established that typhoid was transmitted by feces and could be reliably prevented with adequate sewers and clean food and water, but most practicing physicians still did not believe that typhoid was a bacterial disease. Most held to the conviction that it was caused by poisons in the water or in the air.[76] Miasms were hard to get rid of.

Even though Woodward's "typho-malarial fever" had been put to rest, malaria and typhoid continued to be confused. Part of that had to do with the fact that typhoid transmission by flies had yet to be proven. A variety of theories were put forward to explain the apparent lack of transmission including the idea that harmless intestinal bacteria could, when exposed to rotting organic matter, morph into typhoid.[77]

Even though the etiology of typhoid remained in doubt, the diagnosis itself could be made with certainty by the time the Spanish war started. In 1896 Ferdinand Widal had shown that, when serum from a suspected typhoid patient was dripped into a culture of typhoid bacilli in bouillon and incubated at 37° Celsius for two or three hours, the typhoid bacteria clumped together and sank to the bottom of the flask leaving clear medium. The test could even be done with a single drop of serum under a microscope. William Osler found the Widal test 95.5 percent positive in typhoid cases and 98.4 percent negative in those without the disease.[78] But Army surgeons had neither laboratories nor microscopes, and almost all relied on their inconsistent clinical acumen to make the diagnosis.

In 1898 the cause of typhoid had been found, an accurate diagnostic test had been developed, and the means to prevent an epidemic were known. And it made no difference.

Newspaper reports and letters home caused predictable public outrage. At that point, Walter Reed entered the story. We will spend more time on Reed when we get to yellow fever, but for now suffice it to say that Sternberg appointed him and Majs. Victor Vaughan and Edward Shakespeare of the volunteer Army to inspect the camps. Reed, the only regular Army officer of the three, chaired the commission.

Their 2,600-page report was scathing. Every regiment they inspected had typhoid, although Army surgeons had correctly diagnosed only about half of them. Ambulatory typhoid cases interacted freely with the uninfected, and contaminated clothing, bedding, and feces were not sterilized. The board recognized the importance of asymptomatic carriers and placed blame for the disaster squarely on officers who had ignored Sternberg's recommendations. In a final report they concluded that, "camp pollution was the greatest sin committed by the troops in 1898."[79]

President William McKinley, acutely aware of the epidemic's political consequences, appointed the War Investigating Commission chaired by railroad executive Maj. Gen. Grenville Dodge to look at the food, clothing, housing, and medical care received by the volunteers. The Dodge Commission was mostly political theater, but it did result in the reform of the Medical Bureau and regulations making officers directly responsible for the health of their men. Clean water, clean food, and clean bodies became military essentials, and military surgeon and historian P. M. Ashburn said in 1909, "it is not probable that the evil conditions of the camps of 1898 will ever be repeated in camps of the regular army."[80] It took two wars for the Army to learn camp sanitation, and typhoid was never a serious problem again for the American military. But Ashburn did not reckon with airborne epidemics.

A DIFFERENT APPROACH TO ECOLOGY

Mosquitoes, Microbes, and Medics

The experience with epidemics in the Spanish-American War is two separate stories with quite different outcomes. We have seen the tragedy of camp typhoid. Yellow fever was a triumph.

THE DISEASE

Flaviviridae (literally yellow viruses) are a family of about seventy mostly arthropod-borne RNA viruses that reproduce by commandeering the endoplasmic reticulum manufacturing system in the cytoplasm of host cells. The yellow fever RNA is a relatively simple 10,233-unit single nucleotide chain that encodes only three structural and three nonstructural proteins. The structural proteins form new virus while the nonstructural ones stay behind to drive more protein production. After the new building blocks are formed, they come together and co-opt a two-layer lipid outer coat from the host's cell membrane before escaping into the bloodstream to infect new cells.

Yellow fever is carried from human to human by the female *Aedes* (formerly called *Stegomyia*) *aegypti* mosquito, a domesticated insect that lays its eggs in shallow pools of fresh water common to an urban environment—cisterns, tin cans, gutters, old tires, and fragments of broken pottery. The mosquito can survive on sugar alone, but the females require blood protein to ovulate.[1] A fertile female will lay about one hundred eggs three times in its two-week lifespan. *Aedes aegypti* are homebodies, generally staying close to the ground and rarely traveling more than three hundred meters from where they are born unless they hitch a ride on a traveling victim. The virus takes up residence in the mosquito salivary glands; virus and insect coexist so perfectly that one might consider the insect the primary host. In a sense, humans are only convenient transportation.

A female *Aedes* can ingest two to three times its body weight in blood in ninety seconds, and three days later she can transmit the virus to a new human host. Virus on the insect *proboscis* initially invades the dendritic cells of the human epidermis where it starts to proliferate. After that there is a range of clinical presentations.

Some cases are subclinical, causing little more than a flu-like illness. In others after an incubation period of three to six days, clinical yellow fever explodes. The "period of infection" reflects release of the virus into the bloodstream and is characterized by the sudden onset of fever, chills, and

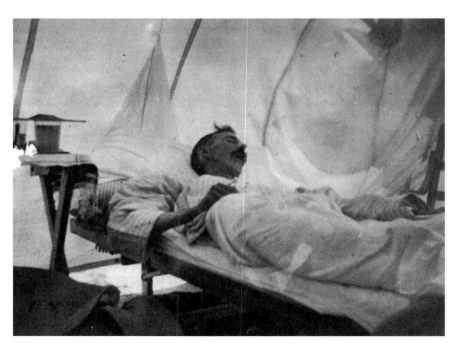

Yellow fever patient in a hospital in Siboney, Cuba *National Library of Medicine*

headache. Over the next three to four days victims develop severe headaches and photophobia, muscle and backaches, nausea, vomiting, irritability, and dizziness. The skin and conjunctivae become congested, and the swollen liver is tender to palpation. The temperature spikes from 102° to 105° with the higher levels being a particularly ominous sign.

The period of infection is followed by a period of remission—the eye of the hurricane. The fever and the symptoms abate, and many patients simply recover. About one in seven, however, progress to the period of intoxication forty-eight hours later. Fever, nausea, and vomiting recur, and multiple organs fail. Protein appears in the urine, renal output drops, blood pressure and pulse become unstable, and the heart enlarges. Liver damage causes epigastric pain and jaundice, and blood fails to clot when the organ stops producing coagulation factors. Gums bleed, and the victim vomits black "coffee grounds" of broken-down blood from the stomach and upper intestines. Thick black stools come from bleeding in the distal bowel, and blood appears in vaginal discharge. The skin turns purple and red from bruises and petechiae, and venipuncture sites bleed. Agitation, delirium, seizures, and coma accompany central nervous system involvement, although that is most often from metabolic abnormalities rather than direct infection of the brain, which is rare.

Between the fifth and tenth day the patient either recovers or dies. Reported case fatality rates vary widely, but about 20 percent of those with jaundice do not survive. There is still no effective treatment for yellow fever.

After its original outbreaks for reasons that are unclear but may reflect widespread immunity among survivors, yellow fever seemed to disappear after it was first brought to the Western Hemisphere by the first European settlers. Sadly the respite was temporary; new cases came on slave ships, and military expeditions brought a recurring supply of non-immunes.

YELLOW FEVER IN THE WESTERN HEMISPHERE

To understand what happened in Cuba in 1898 it is necessary to remember the dire influence of yellow fever around the Caribbean and up the eastern coast of the United States for the preceding two and a half centuries.

Great Britain claimed the island of Barbados in 1625 and built its first settlement there in 1627. Sugar cane was brought from Dutch Brazil a few years later and was followed almost immediately by slave ships from Africa. Yellow fever came in 1647. Genetic sequencing suggests that the virus had been present in West Africa for three thousand years, but Caribbean sugar plantations provided a perfect environment for the *Aedes* mosquito that carried the pathogen. Neither the virus nor the mosquitoes stayed in Barbados; yellow fever was described in a Mayan manuscript the following year.[2] During the ensuing decades epidemics killed more than a quarter of the population of Barbados, Guadeloupe, St. Kitts, Cuba, the Yucatán, and the Caribbean coast of Central America.[3]

European military expeditions in the Caribbean fared poorly. It only took a week in May 1655 for seven thousand British troops to seize Jamaica during the Anglo-Spanish War. By November 47 percent of that force was dead, and half the survivors were sick. Yellow fever, malaria, and less well-defined fevers took 20 percent of the garrison every year, about seven times the mortality rate of British soldiers stationed in Canada.

In 1689, a British invasion of Guadeloupe failed when half the troops that went ashore died of disease. Three years later the Royal Navy tried again and lost half their crews to yellow fever. The experience was repeated in Martinique in 1693. During the War of the Leagues of Augsburg (1688–97), a combined British and Spanish force lost 60 percent of its men to disease in a failed attempt to take Saint-Domingue. In the War of the Spanish Succession (1701–13), French and British forces attacked Spain in the Americas nineteen times, but these expeditions were thwarted at least fourteen and perhaps eighteen times by disease. During the War of Jenkins' Ear and the War of the Austrian Succession (1739–48), Admiral Edward Vernon took Portobello and Chagres in Central America and tried to take Cartagena. He lost 41 percent of his men, only 650 of whom died from wounds. He gave up and tried to take Santiago, Cuba, on his return voyage. That cost him three-quarters of the men he had left, only one thousand from wounds and the rest to yellow fever.

In 1762, during the Seven Years' War (1754–63), Admiral George Pocock's 14,000 men laid siege to Havana. Almost as soon as the men landed they were attacked by yellow fever. Within a few months, 4,708 died from disease while only 255 were lost in combat. In mid-1763, the British gave up and returned Havana to Spain having lost more men in thirteen months in Cuba than in the rest of the North American campaigns in the Seven Years' War combined.

In 1780, a British expeditionary force tried to take Fort San Juan in Nicaragua, but fevers killed 77 percent of the men and the effort failed. One of the lucky survivors was twenty-one-year-old Royal Navy lieutenant Horatio Nelson.

Perhaps the most significant impact of yellow fever in the Americas resulted from the 1791 slave revolt in Saint-Domingue (currently Haiti and the Dominican Republic). In 1794, the British occupied major ports on the island to reverse the revolt and lost 50,000 men, mostly to yellow fever, before giving up. The island had been the richest source of sugar income in the Caribbean and had been the source of about half the tropical produce sent to Europe, occupying over 1,000 ships and 15,000 sailors.

In 1802, French First Consul Napoleon Bonaparte, anxious to recover the income lost to the Haitian revolt and imagining a new American colonial empire based on Caribbean sugar and French control of the Mississippi River, dispatched his brother-in-law General Charles Victor Emmanuel Leclerc and 60,000 troops to Saint-Domingue. Yellow fever won that campaign as well; Leclerc and 50,000 of his troops died on the island, and Bonaparte lost interest in his American empire. When President Thomas Jefferson sent Robert Morris and James Monroe to Paris with an offer to either lease or buy the port of New Orleans, Napoleon's representative offered to sell not just New Orleans but the entire Louisiana territory for $15 million or about $18 per square mile.[4]

YELLOW FEVER AND THE UNITED STATES

Yellow fever epidemics were not confined to the Caribbean. In the eighteenth century, New York City saw fifteen epidemics, Charleston twelve, Boston eight, and Baltimore seven. There were major outbreaks in Mobile, Norfolk, Galveston, Pensacola, Natchez, and Key West as well. Philadelphia had perhaps the worst of all in a 1793 epidemic that may have come with a shipload of refugees from the Saint Domingue revolt. The true numbers are unknown, but it is likely that more than five thousand people—about one-tenth of the city's population—died of yellow fever in Philadelphia that year. The United States had ample reason to fear the disease.

There was a short respite, but yellow fever returned with a vengeance in the second half of the 1800s. One reason for the recurrence was a smoldering rebellion in Cuba that flared into a Ten Years' War (1868–78). The revolt was put down, but not before tens of thousands of refugees fled to the United States. The worst epidemic in more than a century started in the city of New Orleans, likely sparked by the arrival of a ship from Havana that evaded quarantine. The city eventually had 25,000 cases, but New Orleans was only the beginning. The epidemic spread to adjoining towns and then up the Mississippi River, ultimately striking 132 towns and cities with 120,000 cases and more than 20,000 deaths. Disruption of local business and trade cost at least $100 million and possibly twice that much.

Closing the border to Cubans was ineffective. Fishermen, smugglers, and refugees continued to come ashore along the Gulf of Mexico avoiding quarantine stations. By 1892, it was estimated that as many as 100,000 people a year moved back and forth between the island and the United States.

One of the most popular places for smugglers to land was near the Gulf Coast resort town of Ocean Springs, and returning vacationers brought the disease to New Orleans in 1897. That epidemic lasted two months with 1,700 cases, two hundred deaths, and devastating social and economic disruption. Railroad traffic for three hundred miles around the city stopped, and cities as far apart as Jackson and Galveston banned people coming from New Orleans. When Atlanta agreed to take refugees from New Orleans, Chattanooga, Charleston, Wilmington, and cities across Alabama banned travel from that city. The U.S. mint in New Orleans stopped coining money because it was assumed to be contaminated and could not be moved out of the city. Business came to a halt, and the New York Stock exchange swooned.

Between 1700 and 1900 the United States suffered through almost one hundred yellow fever epidemics, and many if not most could be traced to Cuba. The chairman of the House Committee on Industry and Commerce warned President William McKinley that Cuba, and especially Havana, posed an unacceptable threat to the health and economic well-being of the country.

In 1898, the United States was a first-rate economic and industrial power with a third-rate navy and a fourth-rate army. Great Britain, France, and the Netherlands had empires, Germany was acquiring one, and Spain was struggling to hold onto the remains of its own. One of those Spanish remnants was less than one hundred miles from the United States that had coveted it for most of the century. Yellow fever was an excuse to take Cuba, a danger if it was not taken, and a way for the fledgling American Army to make its reputation.

NINETEENTH-CENTURY MEDICINE

Medicine in the United States at the end of the nineteenth century was ill-equipped to cope with epidemic yellow fever. Illness was classified by symptoms rather than cause, and epidemics were lumped together and thought to be "a putridity or fermentation of the blood, and gastric and intestinal hemorrhages" and were "like the skin eruptions, sweats and abscesses, regarded as conservative efforts on the part of the system to rid itself of decomposed material resulting from this fermentation of the blood."[5] Black vomit, the hallmark of yellow fever, was thought to be expulsion of decomposed liver cells.

It was obvious to eighteenth-century Philadelphia physician Benjamin Rush that red, tachypneic, sweating, febrile patients suffered from an excess of blood, so he removed as much as a quarter of it to restore balance. He added mercury-containing calomel to promote salivation as well as emetics and purgatives to get rid of excess gastrointestinal humors. That any of his patients survived is more a testament to their fortitude than their therapy, but Rush's "heroic" regime persisted well into the following century.

Medical training ignorant of the cause of infectious disease was of limited use, and medicine's scientific and practical deficiencies were on full display in mid-nineteenth century America. Most practitioners had minimal classroom training and no exposure to a laboratory. What clinical medicine they knew was gleaned from apprenticeships.

On the positive side, physicians had largely abandoned the idea that disease resulted from divine intervention or humoral imbalance. Many were looking for more rational explanations and had become astute observers of local conditions. It was clear that, at least in temperate climates, yellow fever was seasonal. It favored warm, moist areas, especially ports where organic products (coffee, tropical fruits) were left to rot. A decomposing mass of coffee left on Philadelphia's docks was blamed for the 1793 epidemic. Port cities were also liable to have unpaved roads running with raw sewage that settled and accumulated at the bottom of shallow bays. Havana was notorious for being smelled before it could be seen.

It was obvious to the observant nineteenth-century physician that yellow fever was caused by miasms emanating from rotting organic matter aggravated by a hot, wet climate. The solution was obvious as well. "Docks or other localities liable to be visited by the disease, courts, yards, gutters, cellars should be left perfectly clear; all accumulations of filth and stagnant water should be carefully removed; streets, courts, and alleys should be paved."[6] If filth caused the disease sanitation was the answer, and vast sums were spent cleaning up polluted cities. That may well have lessened the incidence of dysentery, typhoid, and cholera, but it did nothing to alleviate yellow fever.

Yellow fever did not spread from skin-to-skin contact like smallpox, but it had most of the other characteristics of contagion. Perhaps the disease was transmitted from person to person by "fomites," tiny particles of contagion clinging to clothes and bedding of the sick. The profuse blood, vomitus, diarrhea, and sweat from dying patients were obvious, and the fomite theory held on tenaciously through the nineteenth century.

Although his work was ignored, the fomite theory had been disproven in dramatic fashion by medical student Stubbins Ffirth in 1802. Working from the observation that direct person-to-person transmission of yellow fever did not resemble that in measles and smallpox, Ffirth set out to eliminate contagion as a source of yellow fever altogether. First he tried to cause the disease in a variety of animals by exposing them to or injecting them with material from yellow fever patients. When that failed to cause disease he began experiments on himself. Ffirth put black vomit under his skin. His arms became inflamed, but the wounds healed and he did not get yellow fever. He tried blood, saliva, sweat, urine, and bile the same way without causing the disease. He heated the vomit and inhaled the steam and drank what was left behind. There was still no yellow fever, and Ffirth concluded that the excreta of yellow fever patients contained nothing that would transmit the disease. The fomite theory should have been put to rest, but practitioners ignored him. Fomites hung around for another hundred years.

If contagion was the problem quarantine should have been the answer, but clearly it was not. In 1896 Dr. Alvah Doty concluded, "A careful investigation shows that quarantine, as a means of controlling the outbreaks referred to (yellow fever) has not been as successful as we could wish, although carried out in a most rigid manner. . . . Therefore, we are stimulated to look for some other means of securing the desired result."[7]

There was another theory about yellow fever spreading. In 1807, Dr. John Crawford of Baltimore wondered if malaria, yellow fever, and possibly other diseases were caused by the mosquitoes that were so much more common in fever season and in the swampy locales that fever seemed to favor, but he went no farther than conjecture. In 1848, Mobile gynecologist Dr. Josiah Nott raised the same question after losing four of his children to yellow fever.[8] He believed yellow fever was a distinct disease unrelated to intermittent, remittent, or pernicious fevers or to commonly diagnosed typho-malarial fever. Moreover it was unlikely to be transmitted in the air. Perhaps the animalcules visible under a microscope could fly from place to place like visible insects and cause disease where they are lit. Nott said, "We can well understand how Insects wafted by the winds (as happens with mosquitoes, flying ants, many of the *Aphides*, etc.) should haul up on the first tree, house, or other object in their course, offering a resting place; but no one can imagine how a gas or emanation, entangled or not with aqueous vapor, while sweeping along on the wings of the wind could be caught in this way."[9] Nott was, however, more poetic than correct.

Louis-Daniel Beauperthuy, a French physician working in Venezuela in 1853, posited a relation between mosquitoes and malaria and yellow fever based on the seasonal coincidence of the insect and the diseases, but he guessed that the mosquito picked up a toxin from decaying organic matter and injected it when it bit a human victim. He was close to the truth but not quite there.

The microscope was the key to a new understanding of infection. Exploring fermentation and spoilage in wine and milk, French scientist Louis Pasteur demonstrated that airborne microorganisms rather than "spontaneous generation" caused the underlying chemical change that either created or destroyed agricultural products. It was a short step to the conclusion that those same organisms could cause human disease. When Pasteur showed that he could weaken the bacteria that caused cholera in chickens, inoculate susceptible poultry with the new strain, and produce immunity much like Jenner's vaccine for smallpox, controlling infection seemed imminent. His rabies vaccine came soon after, and the race was on to find other explainable and controllable diseases. Johns Hopkins physician and historian Howard Kelly said, "Medicine, both as a science and an art, had entered upon a new era, already rich in achievement and still richer in promise."[10]

After yellow fever tracked up the Mississippi River in 1878 it was obvious to most observers that yellow fever traveled, and it was probably caused by a microorganism. The bug just had to be found. During last two decades of the nineteenth century, putative causative organisms were discovered and dismissed dozens of times.

YELLOW FEVER AND THE ARMY

The stage was now set for another scientific and therapeutic revolution, and physicians in the U.S. Army Medical Service were the revolutionaries. That story begins with George Miller Sternberg.

Sternberg graduated from the College of Physicians and Surgeons at Columbia University in the spring of 1860 and practiced briefly in New Jersey before taking the examination to join the Army Medical Corps. He finished last of twenty applicants, but the Civil War had started, and the Union Army needed every physician it could find, so Sternberg was commissioned and assigned to the Army of the Potomac in May 1861.[11]

After the war Sternberg stayed in the Army and published two papers on the "poison" of yellow fever and its natural history in the *New Orleans Medical and Surgical Journal*, which launched his reputation as an expert in the disease. In 1879, Sternberg was brought back to Washington and assigned to the Havana Yellow Fever Commission of the National Board of Health charged with investigating the cause and control of the disease and the relation of the 1878 epidemic to Cuba.

The commission spent that summer in Havana, and in August the Spanish governor of Cuba assigned Dr. Carlos Finlay to work with them.[12]

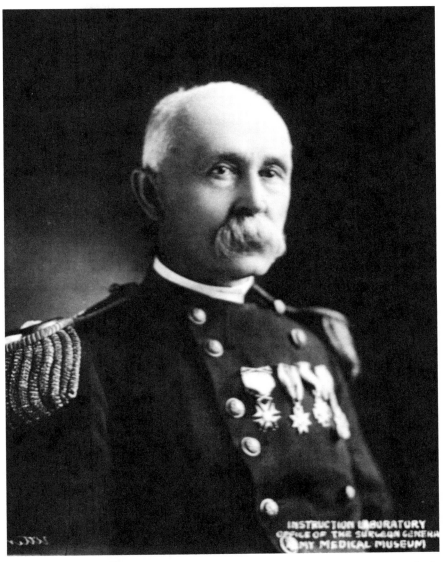

Surgeon General George Sternberg ordered the investigations that led to control of yellow fever in Cuba. *National Library of Medicine*

Finlay was an erudite, modest, kind man with a wide-ranging intellect whose interests included physics, chemistry, mathematics, meteorology, history, and languages. He spoke Spanish, French, German, and English and read Latin and Greek, but his passion was yellow fever.

Havana was probably the best place in the world to study yellow fever. In most places the disease was seasonal, but it was not in Cuba. In the 408 months between 1856 and 1879 there was only one month in which yellow fever had not been documented. The disease was so pervasive the commission was sure it was in the air. Finlay went further, concluding that yellow fever had to be carried from an infected person to a susceptible one by "an agent whose existence is entirely independent of the disease and the diseased."[13]

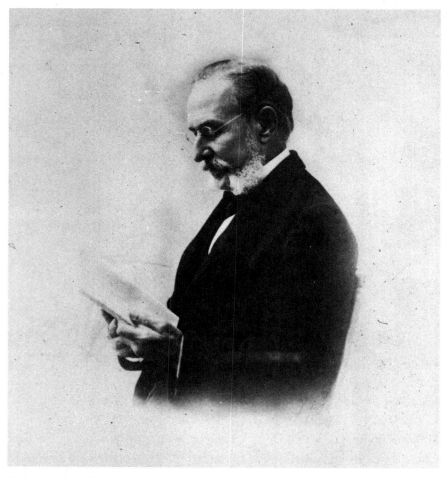

Cuban epidemiologist Carlos Finlay long suspected yellow fever was transmitted by mosquitoes but could not prove it. *National Library of Medicine*

He settled on mosquitoes as that agent and claimed he had transmitted the disease to five people by having them bitten. His evidence was hardly conclusive. First there was question about whether the subjects actually caught the disease. Besides they lived in areas where yellow fever was endemic, so there was no certainty mosquitoes were the cause even if they carried yellow fever. The paper was met with deafening silence, and Finlay spent the next nineteen years doing 104 experiments trying to prove he was right.

Although the fomite theory still had many adherents among clinicians, microbiologists were convinced a microorganism caused yellow fever. They just had to find it. Groups from Philadelphia, Paris, and Panama among others claimed to have found the organism, and Sternberg spent the rest of his research career investigating and disproving those claims.

Sternberg's old acquaintance Carlos Finlay was among those who proposed a causative organism. He cultured what he called *Micrococcus tetragenus febris flavus* from mosquitoes that had fed on yellow fever patients, but cultures he sent to Sternberg proved to be contaminated with a variety of organisms and unrelated to yellow fever. Finlay may have been "a most enthusiastic and industrious investigator," but he was no microbiologist.

During a trip to Mexico, Sternberg proposed an experiment. He said, "If the infectious agent of yellow fever is present in the blood, we would expect that the disease may be transmitted by inoculating a susceptible person with blood drawn from one sick with the disease. Dr. Finlay, of Havana, believes that the disease is commonly transmitted by mosquitoes, which, after filling themselves from a yellow fever patient, transmit the germ by inoculation into susceptible persons." Experimental inoculation would be "the most satisfactory and direct way of determining whether the infectious agent is present in the blood."[14] Sternberg told his wife that such an experiment—a challenge trial—would not be ethically possible in the United States, but he found a physician in Vera Cruz who was already doing something similar.

In 1885, Dr. Daniel Ruiz injected blood and urine from a yellow fever patient into an "unacclimated" subject but failed to reproduce the disease. He agreed to repeat the experiment for Sternberg. His first two subjects were injected with blood from a patient whose yellow fever diagnosis was

questionable, but the third donor clearly had the disease. Fifty cubic cen-
timeters (cc) of blood were drawn and injected subcutaneously into the
experimental subject. (That seems an enormous amount to put under the
skin but it is what Sternberg reported.) Again no yellow fever developed,
and Sternberg surmised that the donor had already begun to recover. He
was anxious to try again, but his time in Mexico had ended, and he was
ordered back to the United States.

Sternberg later said that, had the Ruiz inoculation succeeded, it
"would have led inevitably to the conclusion that yellow fever, like malarial fever, is transmitted by an intermediate host, and that this intermediate
host is a mosquito."[15] For the rest of his life Sternberg remained convinced
that only bad luck had kept him from the credit that ultimately went to
Walter Reed.

In 1893, Sternberg was named surgeon general of the Army and promoted brigadier general. One of the first things he did on returning to
Washington was to establish an Army Medical School to teach freshly
trained physicians to be military surgeons. They were taught how to site
buildings based on ventilation and drainage, how to dispose of sewage and
garbage, and how to provide safe food and water by disinfection of slaugh-
terhouses, kitchens, and mess halls. Sternberg was essentially training sanitary engineers, but his students also learned bacteriology, microscopy, and
urine analysis along the way.

At the same time, Congress reduced the number of Army assistant
surgeons from 125 to 110 and replaced the contract surgeons with private
practitioners paid on a fee-for-service basis. It was an interesting decision
since those serving in the Medical Corps were better trained and more
carefully selected than the private practitioners who replaced them.

While that was going on, medical education underwent a seminal
change much of which took place in Baltimore. Thanks to a generous
endowment Johns Hopkins University was on the cusp of revolutioniz-
ing medical education. The trustees planned to build a new hospital and
integrate it with a four-year medical school. The school would admit only
those with undergraduate degrees, and the entire faculty would be full-
time employees engaged in not just education but in clinical practice and
basic research as well.

Hopkins' intention had never been to train practitioners. The school was built to train educators, and the men and women from its programs created new specialties and started academic programs from New England to California.

The Hopkins hospital was finished in 1889, but much of the medical school endowment was in Baltimore and Ohio Railroad stock that fared poorly in the post–Civil War depression. As a result the school did not open until 1893, just when Sternberg came to Washington. Hopkins, and especially Howard Welch's laboratory, were to have a profound effect on the Army Medical Service beginning with Walter Reed.

Reed was the youngest of five children of an impoverished Methodist minister in Gloucester County in far eastern Virginia. His mother died when Walter was only fourteen, and the boy enrolled at the University of Virginia the following year. The university waived its sixteen-year-old minimum age requirement since Reed's older brother Christopher was already a student with the stipulation that the two room together. In 1867, Reed studied Latin, Greek, and English literature, but at the end of that academic year his father told him he did not have the resources to send the two boys and their older brother for full undergraduate educations simultaneously.

Medicine took less time and less money, so Reed transferred the following year. His medical studies lasted only from October 1868 to the end of June the following year. There were forty-nine in that year's University of Virginia graduating class, ten of whom received medical degrees. Reed graduated third of the ten and remains, at age seventeen, the youngest to ever graduate from the medical school at Charlottesville.

After graduation and additional training in New York, Reed intended to start a private practice to supplement his income, but he had two strikes against him. He was not from New York, so he had no social connections. Besides, although he was strikingly handsome, he looked even younger than his twenty-two years and did not engender the confidence necessary to attract patients. Reed needed an alternative, and three or four years in the U.S. Army looked to be a good solution.

First he had to pass the notoriously difficult examination for a Medical Service commission. The best description of the examination is by Albert Truby who was examined by Reed himself a few years later. The

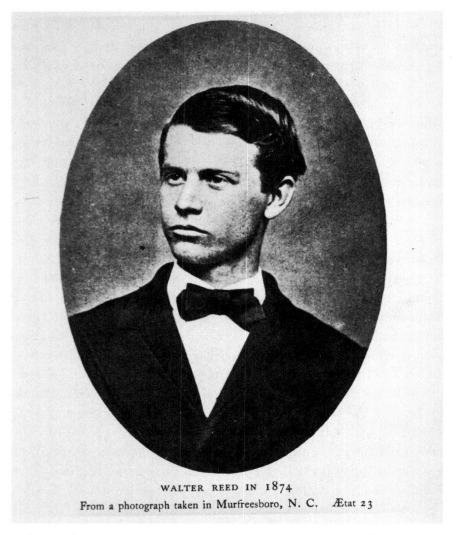

WALTER REED IN 1874
From a photograph taken in Murfreesboro, N. C.   Ætat 23

Walter Reed as a young man. His boyish good looks made it impossible to build a private practice and led to his joining the Army Medical Corps. *National Library of Medicine*

test changed little in the interim.[16] When Reed took the examination, five hundred applicants competed for thirty available slots. The first hurdle was a thorough physical examination that eliminated about a third of the hopefuls. Those that passed faced thirty hours of written and oral tests spread over five days. The candidates had to demonstrate proficiency in classical languages, mathematics, and history before even starting on medicine. Failure of any section resulted in immediate dismissal. Ironically, one of Reed's written questions was on the spread and control of yellow fever. He said the disease was caused by germs that clung to clothes and cargo or by exposure to a sick patient and that control relied on rigorous sanitation.

Reed passed despite being told that his knowledge of literature and science was less than that expected of an Army surgeon. On July 2, 1875, he was granted a commission "equivalent" to a first lieutenancy and became number 112 of the 120-member Medical Corps.

Reed had fifteen assignments over the next eighteen years, mostly in Western forts where he was the general physician to soldiers and their families as well as miscellaneous civilians and local Indians. Wounds, venereal disease, and alcoholism were the bulk of his practice, but he got a brief respite early in 1881 when he was assigned to Fort McHenry in Baltimore. He took advantage of the opportunity to attend physiology lectures at Johns Hopkins. He was not there long enough to take formal courses, but it was his first taste of academic medicine. In 1889, after another series of western postings, Reed requested a three-month leave to take "the opportunity of pursuing certain special studies in my profession."[17] Although he had risen to the rank of major Reed was thirty-nine years old, and his career had stalled. He was granted the leave with one stipulation: the surgeon general instructed him to only take courses that bore directly on his clinical duties as an Army surgeon. Besides, three months was not enough for what Reed had in mind. Although Hopkins would not open its medical school for another three years, the hospital was functioning and teaching formal courses in bacteriology and pathology. Unfortunately for Reed those courses ran for seven months.

Luckily Jedidiah Hyde Baxter became Army surgeon general in 1890. He granted Reed three months' leave and managed to have him assigned as examiner of recruits in Baltimore after that. The Army surgeon worked under Welch from October 1889 to October 1890 and became a research scientist. Welch was impressed with his technical skill and hard work, and he allowed Reed to both share in his own research and to work independently.

Reed's life changed dramatically in 1893 when Sternberg became surgeon general and established the Army Medical School. The surgeon general did not have the funds to recruit outside faculty, so he staffed the school with active-duty physicians. Reed was appointed Professor of Clinical and Sanitary Microscopy and taught urine analysis and bacteriology. He was also made curator of the Army Medical Museum, succeeding John Shaw Billings who had been instrumental in starting the Johns Hopkins Medical School.

Now teaching and research occupied all his time. Although Reed had never taught, he genuinely enjoyed the students, and he took a second appointment teaching bacteriology at Columbian Medical School (later George Washington University Medical School). The students found him entertaining and informative, although his voice drifted into an irritating falsetto when he got excited. In the following years Reed studied and wrote about rabies (including a paper co-authored with Sternberg), diphtheria antitoxin, erysipelas, typhoid, malaria, and yellow fever. The frontier Army physician became a recognized expert in infectious disease.

Reed maintained contact with Hopkins and acquired an associate who also trained there. James Carroll was tall, thin, and pale with rapidly receding red hair. Born in England, he emigrated to Canada at age fifteen. Carroll drifted from job to job living as a backwoodsman on the Canadian frontier until 1874 when he wandered across the border and joined the U.S. Army as a hospital steward, a job that could make one an orderly, pharmacist, or clerk. Carroll liked the assignment, took an interest in medicine, and—with some difficulty—secured permission to attend medical lectures in St. Paul, Minnesota. Over the next few years he added courses at Bellevue and the University of Maryland where he finally received a medical degree in 1891.

Carroll took graduate courses in bacteriology at Johns Hopkins in the winters of 1891–92 and 1892–93 after which he was assigned to the Army Medical Museum as Reed's assistant. Welch later noted how often Reed and Carroll were together at Hopkins lectures and presentations, but the relationship between Reed and Carroll was, according to Reed's friend Jefferson Kean, not a close one. "Carroll came to Reed's office as an enlisted man, half educated and not of social standing in the Army

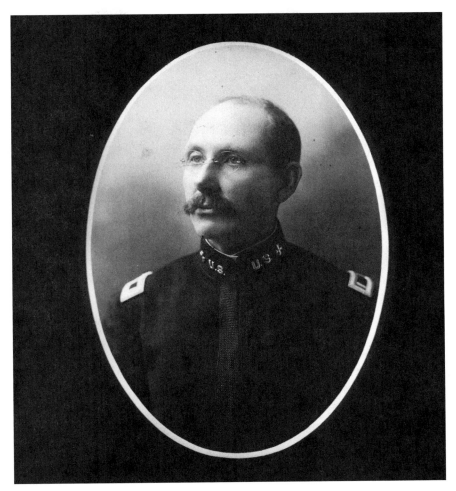

U.S. Army physician James Carroll was instrumental in the yellow fever experiments in Cuba. *National Library of Medicine*

and he never entirely was of the same social standing with Reed and his friends."[18]

Kean was interesting himself. He was born in Lynchburg, Virginia, a descendant of John Rolfe and the great-grandson of Thomas Jefferson. He graduated from the University of Virginia medical school in 1883, and like Reed went to New York for clinical training but was unable to secure a hospital appointment. He decided to try the military and took the same difficult examination as Reed. He passed second in his group, but there were no available commissions, so he settled for a contract as acting assistant surgeon and was sent to Fort Sill, Oklahoma. From there Kean was transferred to Fort Robinson, Nebraska, where he met Medical Corps Lieutenant Leonard Wood who would be his commanding officer in Havana.

In November 1894 Kean was transferred to Key West. In July 1896, the island saw "a considerable smallpox epidemic," and Reed was sent to investigate. He spent six days staying with the Keans, beginning a friendship that lasted the balance of Reed's life and played a key role in the Cuba yellow fever episode.

Sternberg's preternatural ability to swat down every suggested etiology for yellow fever had quieted the clamor for several years, but there were still researchers anxious to make their careers on the disease. In 1897, two papers purporting to have solved the problem were presented at the Pasteur Institute in Paris. That from Dr. Wolff Havelburg from Rio de Janeiro was quickly put to rest when his organism proved to be a common colon bacillus.

The other candidate was not so easily dismissed. Giuseppe Sanarelli trained at the Pasteur Institute before going to South America as director of the Institute of Experimental Hygiene at the university in Montevideo. In an 1897 article in the *British Medical Journal*, he claimed to have found the bacterium that caused yellow fever. He said he had found his *Bacillus icteroides* in 70–100 percent of autopsied yellow fever cases and had cultured it from 58 percent of patients.

Moreover, Sanarelli claimed to have reproduced yellow fever in multiple animals by injecting his bacteria. He had also injected five patients with filtered cultures from autopsied yellow fever cases and claimed to have reproduced the disease in each although three of the experimental subjects had unfortunately died.

His challenge trials with potentially lethal disease for which there was no treatment were roundly condemned. Victor Vaughn, one of the most prominent bacteriologists in the United States, called the experiment ridiculous. William Osler was more straightforward: "To deliberately inject a poison of known high degree of virulency into a human being, unless you obtain that man's sanction, is not ridiculous, it is criminal."[19] But Osler did not stop there. In a footnote to the entry on yellow fever in his *Principles and Practice of Medicine*, he wrote, "The work of Sanarelli has been marred by a series of unjustifiable experiments upon men, which should receive the unqualified condemnation of the profession . . . if with full knowledge, a fellow creature may submit to certain tests and trials, just as a physician may experiment on himself. . . . But deliberate experiments such as Sanarelli carried out with cultures of known and tested virulence and which were followed by serious, nearly fatal illness, are simply criminal."[20] He set the boundaries of ethical human experimentation—self-experimentation by physicians was acceptable, but experimentation on others was permissible only with explicit and informed consent.

Meanwhile, the question of whether Sanarelli had identified the cause of yellow fever remained undecided. His reputation and the venue where his findings had been presented taken together with a chauvinistic desire to have an Italian conquer what they considered their own disease lent Sanarelli's findings international credibility. But there was still Sternberg who had put forward his own candidate, which he called *Bacillus x* several years earlier and brought back in an 1897 paper with the admission that an etiologic link had not been definitively proven. Sternberg dismissed Sanarelli's organism out of hand. The American had no lack of confidence in his ability as a microscopist, and he sniffed that if the organism had been there he would have seen it.

Sternberg had Reed and Carroll at the Army Medical Museum, and both were teaching and had access to laboratories at Columbian, so he charged them with investigating *B. icteroides*. Reed was inclined to believe Sanarelli, and he and Carroll spent the next year and a half studying his organism. Carroll had experience with hog cholera, a common contaminant in cultures grown in the Caribbean and Central America, and the two eventually concluded that was what Sanarelli had grown. In a short article published in the April 29, 1899, issue of *Medical News* ("*Bacillus icteroides* and *Bacillus cholerae suis*") Reed and Carroll stated that the two organisms were the same and neither had anything to do with yellow fever. Sanarelli's organism was a contaminant.

Four months later, Sanarelli responded in the same journal with a vigorous rebuttal along with personal attacks on Sternberg, Reed, and Carroll.

He said Sternberg was the victim of professional jealousy and was only trying to preserve his own claims. He accused Reed and Carroll of being cal-
low (Sanarelli at thirty-three was five years younger than Reed), provincial,
and without the laboratory or clinical experience of more sophisticated
Europeans. He haughtily suggested that the Americans had "fallen victim
of some deplorable neglect of technical precautions," and had used specimens contaminated with hog cholera. Reed pointed out that the specimens
they used came from the Pasteur Institute and were labeled as having come
from Sanarelli's own Institute of Hygiene.[21]

Besides, Army contract surgeon Aristides Agramonte, who had trained
at Hopkins and worked with Reed, had gone to Santiago during a yellow
fever outbreak and had autopsied ten cases diagnosed with the disease. He
found *B. icteroides* in only three of those, and he concluded that they were
contaminants.

Sanarelli remained famous even after his yellow fever hypothesis was
proven false and was nominated for the Nobel Prize in Physiology or Medicine in 1937 for his work on infectious enteropathies and immunology of
tuberculosis.

THE SPANISH-AMERICAN WAR

While the Sanarelli conflict raged an actual war broke out. The United
States had flirted with annexing Cuba for most of the nineteenth century. The island was fertile, well populated, a major source of agricultural
exports, and close. An insurrection in Cuba, smoldering for more than
thirty years, flared again in February 1895. Between that year and 1898
the Spanish dispatched thousands of troops, virtually none of whom were
immune to yellow fever, to the island. That force peaked at 230,000 men,
but by 1898 only 55,000 were well enough to fight. Most suffered from one
sort of fever or another (malaria and dysentery being the most common),
and 16,000 had contracted yellow fever.

The Yellow Fever Commission had already concluded that Havana
was a risk to every city of the American South during fever season, and the
situation in Cuba was dire. The Marine Hospital Service sent Surgeon General William Wyman to investigate in May 1895. Wyman's initial report
said there was no immediate danger to the United States, but a flood of

refugees and smugglers avoiding quarantine facilities on the Gulf Coast forced a change of mind.

Southern cities in the United States had been plagued with yellow fever in each of the previous twenty-six years, and Wyman knew that sixteen of those outbreaks could be traced directly to Havana. In 1896, he told attendees at a meeting of the Pan American Medical Congress in Mexico City where he chaired the Committee on International Quarantine that countries in the hemisphere should no longer tolerate the threat from Cuba.[22] U.S. Secretary of State Richard Olney bluntly threatened Spanish Ambassador to the U.S. Enrique Dupuy de Lôme: "Sooner or later the problem of attacking the pestilential conditions which exist and have existed for more than a century at Habana will demand the attention not only of Spain, but of other endangered countries, with a view to devising an effective remedy for the state of things disclosed in Surgeon-General Wyman's report, and the gravity of the situation invites timely attention and action."[23]

Concern escalated in September 1897 when yellow fever broke out in Louisiana and Mississippi. The yellow press had a field day. In September 1897, William Randolph Hearst's *New York Journal* said, "The extirpation of Spanish rule in Cuba is a sanitary measure essential to the safety of the United States." The *Houston Daily Post* was more to the point: "If annexing Cuba will result in eradicating yellow fever and quarantine, by all means let us annex it at once."[24]

On February 15, 1898, the U.S. battleship *Maine*, sent to Cuba to intimidate Spain, sank in Havana Harbor, the victim of a massive explosion that claimed the lives of 260 crew members. Although this conclusion has been discredited, on March 28 a U.S. Navy Court of Inquiry found that the ship had been sunk by a Spanish mine.[25] Congress had already allocated $50 million to bolster the pitifully small 26,000-man American army still mostly scattered among small outposts in the West.

On April 20, U.S. Army Commanding General Nelson Miles and Fifth Army Corps commander Maj. Gen. William Shafter told McKinley they could not possibly have 125,000 recruits trained and ready to invade Cuba before June. That would place the invasion at the height of yellow fever season, and Shafter and Miles did not want to wait for the volunteers.

The problem was solved for them when Spain declared war on April 23. The following day Congress voted to declare war and backdated its declaration to April 21. Shafter rushed to collect and arm the 16,000 men of the Fifth Army Corps from the western forts where they were scattered. One volunteer unit was included. The Rough Riders were alliteratively named for Roosevelt although the assistant secretary now lieutenant colonel was second in command to Leonard Wood.

To understand what ensued, it is necessary to spend a bit of time on Wood who had been a military surgeon and White House physician before taking over the First Volunteer Cavalry. He was the son of a Massachusetts family physician and had graduated from Harvard Medical School. Unable to make a living practicing in Boston, Wood took the Army Medical Corps examination in March 1885. Although he finished second out of fifty-nine applicants there was only one commission available, so he started his army career as a $100-a-month contract surgeon.[26]

While posted in San Francisco, Wood met and married the adopted niece of Supreme Court Justice Stephen Field. In 1895, he was transferred to Washington where his wife's relation to Field gave him access to the White House. He became close to President Grover Cleveland who, after losing the 1896 election to William McKinley, advised Wood to stay and care for the new incumbent. That turned out to be surprisingly easy. Ada McKinley was an unabashed hypochondriac, and Wood, muscular and acceptably handsome, became indispensable. He and similarly athletic Assistant Secretary of the Navy Theodore Roosevelt became inseparable.

When the Spanish-American War started Roosevelt and Wood convinced McKinley to let them start their own volunteer cavalry unit. Wood offered to recruit cowboys he had known from Arizona who he promised could ride, shoot, and live off the land. Roosevelt would tap his network of eastern collegiate athletes. When word of the new regiment got out, the two could have filled not just a regiment but an entire division with the flood of applicants. They wound up with "twelve hundred . . . millionaires, paupers, shysters, lawyers, cowboys, quack doctors, farmers, college professors, miners, adventurers, preachers, prospectors, socialists, journalists, insurance agents, Jews, politicians, Gentiles, Mexicans, professed Christians, Indians, West Point graduates, Arkansan wild men, baseball players, sheriffs, and horse thieves."[27] Because he was the one with military experience Wood was named colonel of the regiment with Roosevelt as his second in command, and his medical career was over.

The regular army was not ready for war, even with as weak an opponent as Spain. Neither was the Army Medical Corps. The entire corps had only 177 commissioned officers, although they did bring back fifteen more who had recently been discharged. The surgeon general, six colonels, ten lieutenant colonels, fifty majors, seventy captains, and fifty-five lieutenants were responsible for examining recruits, maintaining sanitation at a string of hastily improvised camps, and learning about tropical diseases while doing general medicine and caring for war wounds.[28]

Each new volunteer regiment was expected to have three medical officers, none of whom were likely to have had military training or experience. A hospital corps was created out of medical students and recent graduates, pharmacists, and whoever was willing to do menial ward work.

Ignorance of tropical disease was not unique to military surgeons. Osler's text said of yellow fever, "The epidemics are invariably due to the introduction of the poison either by patients affected by the disease or through infected articles. Unquestionably the poison may be conveyed by fomites."[29] The Marine Hospital Service's crisp new guide stated, "While yellow fever is a communicable disease it is not contagious in the ordinary acceptation of the term but is spread by the infection of places and articles of bedding, clothing, and furniture."[30] Armed with the most up-to-date medical information, Army Medical Corps physicians fought yellow fever with the wrong tools.

The American invasion of Cuba went better than almost anyone predicted. On June 13, Shafter sailed from Tampa with 819 officers, 16,058 enlisted men, 89 newspaper correspondents, Roosevelt's two moviemakers, and an assortment of clerks, teamsters, stevedores, and foreign observers. The men landed unopposed at Daquiri on Cuba's southeastern coast, and, after a few brief land battles and destruction of the Spanish naval squadron, Brigadier General José Toral surrendered Santiago on July 17.

The city was a reeking mass of garbage, sewage, and rotting animals. On July 13, Miles wired Secretary of War Russell Alger that the health of his troops was in real danger. His army already had one hundred cases of yellow fever and would have half again that many more the next day. Miles assumed the disease emanated from the city's filth.

The troops and their officers worried as well. On August 3, a collection of generals joined by Wood and Roosevelt met and drafted a letter demanding that American soldiers be removed from Cuba as soon as possible. That presented two problems. First Spain had not yet surrendered, and neither Alger nor McKinley wanted Madrid to know how vulnerable the American force was. Second Washington politicians were concerned that returning soldiers would bring yellow fever home with them. Roosevelt, no newcomer to manipulating the press, carefully leaked the Round Robin Letter to the Associated Press. McKinley was furious, but the troops were on the way to Camp Wikoff on the eastern tip of Long Island within three days. In the end there would be 1,575 cases of yellow fever and 231 deaths among American troops in Cuba and none in the United States.[31] But that was not because the troops were quarantined. It was because they did not bring mosquitoes, and Long Island had no resident population of *Aedes*.

The Army still had to deal with Santiago, and the best medical information held that sanitizing the city was the solution. Controlling the population and disinfecting the city were the Army's priorities, and Wood, both a soldier and a physician, looked like the best candidate to do both. On July 20, Wood was given absolute command of a city of some 40,000 people.

What happened next was quite remarkable. During the next six months eighty-five miles of streets were swept with hand-made brooms every day, and 25,000 cubic yards of street trash were gathered up and burned. There was not enough fresh water to wash the streets, so filth was scraped up and 4,000 gallons of carbolic acid and 11,000 pounds of chloride of lime were spread on the residue. Fires fed by 35,000 gallons of petroleum burned 18,000 cubic yards of accumulated garbage. Privies were either emptied with buckets or filled in, and streets were macadamized so sewage could not collect in the mud. The city was clean within a month.

Wood drafted every resident of the city to help. He had control of food supplies, and anyone who wanted to eat worked regardless of social status. People were paid $0.75 a day to work, or $0.50 a day plus rations for one, or nothing and rations for four. A workday was ten hours. Wood spent

$250,000 out of city revenues and made Santiago, which had been reck-oned one of the filthiest cities in the world, one of the cleanest. Any Cuban or Spaniard with a suspicious fever was removed to a quarantine camp a mile across the bay.[32] It was a sanitary triumph.

And it did not stop yellow fever. In August Wood had a severe febrile illness that was never definitively diagnosed although he continued to serve in areas where yellow fever was endemic and never got the disease again, so it is likely he had acquired immunity. At first sanitation seemed to work; yellow fever was apparently gone from Santiago by the fall. But that was really just the end of fever season; the following June an outbreak exploded among Americans in Santiago that included two of Wood's clerks and one of his household staff. The failure of sanitation in Santiago was fresh in Wood's memory when he became governor general of the entire island on January 1, 1900.

The war ended without a clear definition of who held sovereignty; Spanish officials and troops just left. There was no functioning Cuban gov-ernment, and the United States declined ownership of the island. Wood and his staff of unexpectedly talented young technocrats took control and accepted responsibility for the island's myriad problems including yellow fever. The Army Medical Corps was at the forefront of the response.

THE EXPERIMENTS

Reed was sent to Havana in April 1899 to investigate the "electrozone" process for turning seawater into disinfectant and got his first taste of Cuba under American control. The following month Sternberg created yet another commission to study yellow fever and changed Reed's life. This time the board comprised Army surgeons to be headquartered at Camp Columbia, an installation eight miles outside Havana that housed 1,400 American troops. It was formed "for the purpose of pursuing scientific investigation with reference to the infectious diseases prevalent on the island of Cuba and *especially yellow fever*."[33] There was considerable later discussion about whether Sternberg had specifically directed the board to address yellow fever—Reed claimed he had not—or had just sent the board to look at all infectious diseases including leprosy, malaria, and "unclas-sified febrile conditions." Regardless of Reed's recollection it is clear the board was sent to work on yellow fever. Given Sternberg's long pursuit of the yellow fever germ, it is evident he intended Reed to take up the hunt for a cause and finish it.

Reed and Carroll were joined on the yellow fever board by two other Hopkins-trained bacteriologists. Jesse Lazear was a thirty-four-year-old born in Baltimore and raised in western Pennsylvania. He began his undergraduate education at Washington and Jefferson College outside Pittsburgh and earned an undergraduate degree from Johns Hopkins in 1889. After graduating from Columbia's College of Physicians and Surgeons in 1892, Lazear spent a year in Europe with stops at laboratories in Germany, at the Institut Pasteur in Paris, and in Rome where he worked on the relation between malaria and the *Anopheles* mosquito that had been shown to transmit malaria three years earlier by Ronald Ross. Lazear was strikingly handsome with deep-set eyes and a trim Vandyke beard and a generous mustache. Aristides Agramonte described him: "A thorough university man, he was the type of the southern gentleman, kind, affectionate, dignified with a high sense of honor, a staunch friend and a faithful soldier."[34] He was quiet and well liked, and Kean thought him considerably superior to Carroll.

On his return from Europe Lazear was appointed bacteriologist and assistant in clinical microscopy at Hopkins and worked with Osler and Welch who recommended him to Sternberg. When Albert Truby wired Sternberg that his Havana laboratory was overwhelmed by an outbreak of dengue fever, the surgeon general hired Lazear as a contract surgeon and dispatched him to Cuba to help man the laboratory.

The commission's fourth member was Aristides Agramonte. Although he and Lazear had not been close as students, they graduated in the same class from the College of Physicians and Surgeons. Agramonte came from a different background. First he was Cuban, born in Puerto Principe in 1868. His father, Eduardo Agramonte, was a brigadier general in the Cuban insurrection forces and was killed in 1872 after which his family moved to New York City. Agramonte attended the City College of New York and the College of Physicians and Surgeons and graduated with honors in 1892. He sported a handlebar mustache, and almost every photograph shows him with a faraway look, his head tilted back and a bit to the side. Even though

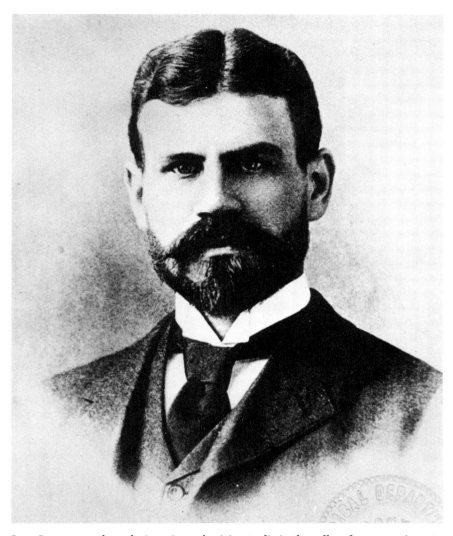

Jesse Lazear was the only American physician to die in the yellow fever experiments.
National Library of Medicine

he had spent all but three years of his life in the United States, the others saw Agramonte as not quite American, and he was never entirely part of the group.

When the war with Spain started Agramonte took a position as a contract surgeon in the Army Medical Corps. His first assignment was to the Army Medical School where he worked with Reed and Carroll on

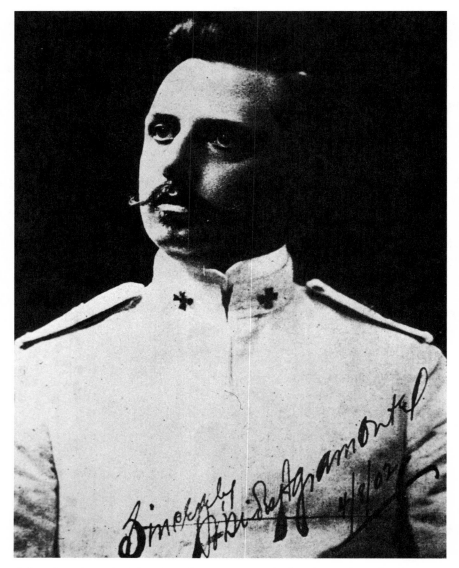

Cuban American physician Aristides Agramonte, the fourth member of Walter
Reed's commission. *National Library of Medicine*

Sanarelli's bacterium. In July 1898, Agramonte was ordered to Santiago to
study yellow fever, probably because he was Cuban and fluent in Spanish.
He was in Cuba again from December 1898 to November 1899 where he
autopsied several cases both with and without yellow fever and concluded

that *Bacillus icteroides* had nothing to do with yellow fever. In May 1900 Agramonte was back in Cuba to take charge of the laboratory at Military Hospital No. 1 and run the hospital's yellow fever ward. On May 25 Sternberg wired him that he had been assigned to Reed's yellow fever board.

Carroll and Reed arrived in Cuba on June 25 to join Lazear and Agramonte. The four men in tropical whites came together for the first time that afternoon on the veranda of the Bachelor Officers Quarters. That meeting was the start of a remarkable cascade of events in which a lethal clinical conundrum that had plagued Western civilization for two and a half centuries was deciphered in two and a half months.

Reed saw his first case of yellow fever the day he arrived—Major Jefferson Randolph Kean, now Chief Surgeon of the Department of Havana. Against specific orders Kean had visited a fellow officer dying from yellow fever. Quarantine restrictions forbade him from entering his friend's sick room, so he sat outside a window and talked to the patient through a grate. Kean later remembered having been bitten by several mosquitoes during the visit. Five days later he had yellow fever, and he nearly died from it. He shrugged off the experience: "I obeyed the letter but not the spirit of the order."[35] Fortunately for Reed the major survived.

Sternberg had directed Reed to report to Wood on arrival in Havana. They estimated that the board's work would take two to three years, and during that time Reed would have to rely on the military governor for supplies and support. Reed and Wood had served at the same time in Western army posts although never together. Because rank in the Medical Corps was a function of length of service, Reed had outranked Wood for a time. Kean and Wood, however, were close and that friendship proved indispensable.

Members of Reed's board began their assignment thinking they were to find the cause of yellow fever in the laboratory, but circumstances dictated otherwise. The month the board came together a yellow fever outbreak in Santa Clara barracks south of Havana resulted in several deaths, and Agramonte was sent to investigate. He and post surgeon J. Hamilton Stone were struck with one case in particular. A trooper contracted yellow fever while in the hospital although the closest case was across a wide yard—clearly too far for a fomite to travel. Agramonte later said he and the

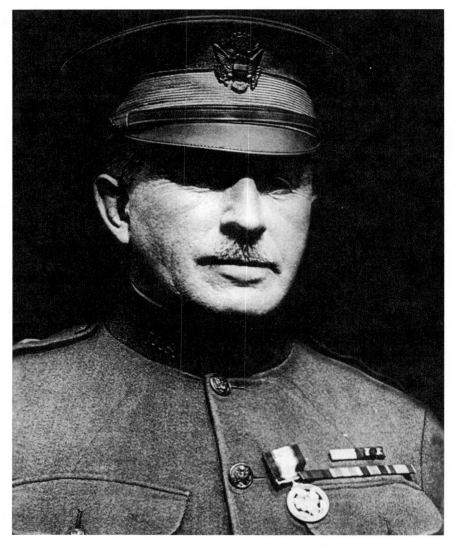

Governor General of Cuba Leonard Wood authorized the yellow fever experiments.
National Library of Medicine

surgeon discussed whether a mosquito might account for the distance the disease had traveled, but they did not follow up on the guess.[36]

The conjecture, however, was not lost. The next month there was another outbreak at a military post in Pinar del Rio 110 miles southwest of Havana. Post surgeons had diagnosed "malarial fever," but Agramonte was again sent to investigate. The day he arrived there was a death, and when he autopsied the patient Agramonte was sure it was yellow fever. When he went on the wards Agramonte found several other cases of "malarial fever" that were clearly misdiagnosed. He said, "a consultation held with the medical officer in charge showed me his absolute incapacity as he was under the influence of opium most of the time."[37] Agramonte strongly suggested that the camp be temporarily abandoned, but the camp commander, unwilling to trade his comfortable barracks for a tent, refused. Agramonte wired Reed who overruled the commander, and the outbreak stopped shortly after the soldiers moved.

Reed harshly criticized the medical staff for missing the correct diagnosis. He and Kean unsuccessfully tried to have the chief surgeon court-martialed, and Reed recommended that all contract surgeons on the base be terminated including newly arrived Robert Cooke. That recommendation was ignored, and Cooke went on to be one of the physician subjects in the yellow fever experiments.

Reed was angry at the medical staff not only for their misdiagnoses but also because they had failed to properly decontaminate clothing and bedding used by the yellow fever patients. He still believed the disease was transmitted by fomites, but there were bothersome anomalies. First the nurses and laundry staff who had surely been exposed to fomites were not getting sick. There was also a worrisome case. Arthur Hoskins, a soldier who had been in the base prison since June 6, came down with yellow fever on July 12.[38] Clearly Hoskins had contracted the disease in jail, but he had shared a cell with eight other men, and none had yellow fever including one who had slept on Hoskins' cot. The best explanation seemed to be that some insect flew into the cell, bit the unfortunate victim, and left without biting anyone else. Reed could not ignore the anomalies. Agramonte said, "It was there on the ground, that for the first time the probability of mosquito agency was seriously discussed by members of the board, and it was decided to carry out some research in this direction."[39]

Reed was finally ready to put the hunt for a causative organism in abeyance while his team investigated how yellow fever was transmitted. Lazear, who had always thought trying to disprove Sanarelli was a waste of time, was delighted. All four commission members knew about Finlay's mosquitoes, and that seemed as good a place to start as any. Since he was the only member of the board experienced with mosquitoes, Lazear was detailed to approach Finlay for the eggs and larvae they needed and to start an *Aedes* breeding program. Finlay was thrilled; at last someone was taking him seriously.

Now the commission's work started in earnest, and, remembering the reaction to Sanarelli's human experiments, the members agreed that the first experiments should be on themselves. Carroll put it this way: "The serious nature of the work decided upon and the risk entailed upon it were fully considered, and we all agreed as the best justification we could offer for experimentation upon others, to submit to the same risk of inoculation ourselves."[40]

Reed conveniently remembered a prior commitment at the Army Medical Museum and returned to Washington before the mosquito experiments began.[41] He later wrote Kean that it was just as well he had not been in Havana to participate in the self-experimentation as "Being an old man, I might have been quickly carried off."[42] He was only three years older than Carroll and five years older than Lazear.

Between August 6 and August 16, Lazear fed his mosquitoes on five infected soldiers. Then he allowed himself to be bitten. All remained in perfect health.

Carroll was skeptical of the mosquito theory, so when he allowed himself to be bitten on August 27 he did not expect to get sick. Lazear administered the bite from a mosquito that had fed on four yellow fever patients twelve days earlier. That was a key piece of luck. Finlay had never transmitted a proven yellow fever case, and the first round of experiments failed to produce the disease because no one realized that there was a delay between the time a mosquito ingested infected blood and when it could transmit the disease. Twelve days was just right.

Carroll was so sure he would not get sick that he went to the yellow fever ward at Las Animas Hospital and even attended an autopsy there after being bitten. He was quite wrong. He became desperately ill as did Private William J. Dean who volunteered to be bitten four days later by the same four mosquitoes plus four more just as Carroll got sick. Dean got yellow fever as well.

Both Dean and Carroll recovered, but Lazear was not so lucky. He probably inoculated both Carroll and Dean and likely felt guilty that he had escaped the disease. What happened next is uncertain. Lazear claimed that he had been accidentally bitten by a mosquito on September 13 while he was on the yellow fever ward, but it is more likely he infected himself. Regardless, this time Lazear got yellow fever and was not as fortunate as Dean and Carroll. By September 22 he was vomiting blood, and three days later he was dead. The telegram to his young wife who had gone home to have a baby simply said, "Doctor Lazear died at eight PM this evening." She did not know he had been ill, and she knew nothing of the experiments that had killed him.[43]

Reed returned to Havana just long enough to write a quick report of what Carroll and Lazear had done. The annual meeting of the American Public Health Association was set for the end of October in Indianapolis, and Sternberg pulled strings to get Reed a last-minute spot on the program to present the findings.

Reed was anxious to get the information out since the Liverpool School of Tropical Medicine had sent Herbert Durham and Walter Myers to America to study yellow fever. During a stop at Havana they met with Reed and Finlay, and, in a September 8 issue of the *British Medical Journal*, wrote that recent discoveries suggested yellow fever was transmitted by mosquitoes. The two had gone on to Brazil where both caught yellow fever and only Durham recovered. Credit for the mosquito theory was at risk.

Reed was upset at Lazear's death but almost as upset with Carroll for leaving the base and contaminating the experiment. To bolster his preliminary Indianapolis report, he needed experiments that were beyond question, and that required facilities and administrative support, so he turned to Wood who had recently been named Cuba's governor general.

Kean took Reed to Wood at an opportune time. In the first place Wood was being judged on his ability to bring order and hygiene to Cuba. He had been deeply disappointed when his sanitation campaign failed to control yellow fever in Santiago, and he had been roundly criticized in the American press for the failure. Worse, yellow fever had broken out in Wood's headquarters. In July forty-eight of his civilian employees and five members of his staff had contracted the disease, and seven of them had died.

When Reed asked for help, Wood was already convinced cleaning the island was not the answer. He offered Reed $10,000 from Cuba's public treasury remarking that he had spent more than that to catch a few thieves who were far less dangerous than yellow fever. Wood directed supply officer Maj. Chauncey Baker to give Reed whatever he needed including tents and equipment that were still in shipping crates and could be presumed uncontaminated. Finally he arranged for Reed to meet with the Spanish consul and secure his approval for enlisting Spanish immigrants as experimental subjects.

Reed later said that the commission's work would not have been possible without Wood's help. Neurosurgeon and Hopkins faculty member Harvey Cushing wrote, "Had the discovery not been made, had one of the soldier-volunteers who contracted the disease (rather than the lamented Lazear, one of the commission) died as a result of the experimental inoculations, one can imagine what a howl would have been raised on the floor of the Senate. . . . Had there not been an intelligent, courageous military governor in Havana willing to take the responsibility for carrying out the experiments, without getting the permission of Congress—well, the Panama Canal would have been an impossibility."[44] Truby concurred; without Wood's approval, "Reed would never have undertaken this dangerous procedure."[45] More than just supplying money and materiel, Wood had taken on himself full responsibility for the experiments and decided without passing it up the chain of command. Agramonte later said, "had a more military and less scientific man been at the head of government, the investigation would have terminated there and then."[46]

Taking responsibility was not without a price. Havana's *La Discusion* headlined "HORRIFIC . . . IF IT'S TRUE. Yellow fever transmitted to Spanish immigrants by mosquitoes!" and went on "a rumor of an act so horrific, repugnant and monstrous has come to us, that hesitating to believe in its existence, almost daring to deny it, we do not hesitate to record it—only by way of rumor—in our columns, because in that way the popular version will arrive directly and quickly to the authorities, and they; if as we hope the deed turns out false, will dispel alarm and if—what we do not believe— it were true, will impose upon its authors exemplary punishment, whose importance is at the height of the monstrous magnitude of the crime."[47]

To keep the experiments clean and to protect the 1,400 non-immune soldiers at Camp Columbia, Reed needed a new facility. Camp Lazear was built at Finca San José, a two-acre farm a few miles west of Havana between Quemados and Marianao that belonged to Agramonte's friend Dr. Ignacio Rojas. The camp was on well-drained soil surrounded by "wild country" and well away from any civilians or even roads.

Camp Lazear began operations on November 20 with a staff of four immunes and nine non-immunes (eight of whom were regular Army soldiers) housed in seven tents. The immunes drove ambulances and supply wagons and assisted with medical treatments. The non-immunes were experimental subjects.

Eventually eleven more Spanish non-immunes were added. Wood, worried about the incidence of yellow fever among recent immigrants, had built a holding camp across the bay from Havana. As each new shipload arrived from Spain, Agramonte was sent to recruit volunteers. They were brought to camp, fed well, and given eight hours a day of light work. Immigrants deemed non-immune who agreed to participate in the experiments were promised $100 in gold with another $100 if they got sick. Once signed up they were not allowed off the grounds of Camp Lazear, and those who did slip out were not allowed back.

In what may have been the first case of written informed consent for a medical experiment, each Spanish participant signed a contract: "The undersigned understands perfectly well that in the case of development of yellow fever in him, that he endangers his life to a certain extent but it being entirely impossible for him to avoid the infection during his stay on this island he prefers to take the chance of contracting it intentionally in the belief that he will receive from the said Commission the greatest care and the most skillful medical service."[48] Of course, "the most skillful medical service" was not worth much in a disease for which there was no effective treatment. Subjects were allowed to assign their payments to whomever they wished if they died.

Two wooden huts were built seventy-five yards from the rest of the camp. Building No. 1, the infected clothing building, was a fourteen-by-twenty-foot wood frame structure built with tongue-and-groove roof and siding impermeable to insects. The building was designed to put to rest once and for all the idea that fomites transmitted yellow fever. The building's only entrance was a solid wooden door leading to a screened vestibule from which a second door opened into the hut. Two south-facing twenty-six-by-thirty-four-inch windows limited air circulation and were shuttered to keep out sunlight that might accidentally decontaminate the building. A wood stove kept the temperature 92–95°F, and the room was constantly damp. It was as tropical as possible.

Bedding and clothes were collected from the yellow fever wards at Las Animas and Camp Columbia, boxed, and held for two weeks to ripen. The linens were soaked with sweat, urine, vomitus, feces, and blood. Initially the stench when they were unpacked was so strong that men who were to stay in the huts ran out gagging and vomiting after only a few minutes, but they eventually returned and unpacked the boxes. Each night the men slept on contaminated sheets wearing contaminated pajamas that they folded and repacked each morning. During the day the men spent their time quarantined in tents. They did that for twenty days.

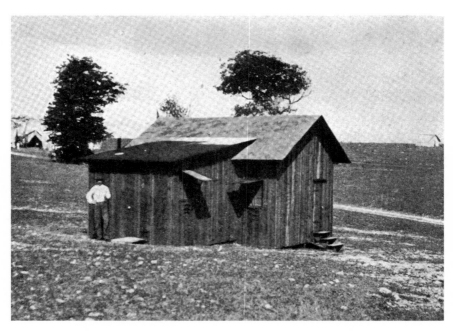

Camp Lazear Building #1, where the initial yellow fever challenge experiments were carried out. *Wellcome Library*

The senior member of the first team was Robert P. Cooke, the youngest doctor at Columbia Barracks. He had attended the U.S. Naval Academy and University of Virginia Medical School before joining the Medical Corps on June 9, 1900. He had just arrived at Pinar del Rio when Agramonte and Reed excoriated the medical staff for misdiagnosing yellow fever. Reed had recommended that Cooke's contract be annulled, but the recommendation was never followed. Cooke and Reed shared a cabin on one of the major's several trips between Washington and Havana, and the two reconciled. Volunteering for the yellow fever experiments was the last step in Cooke's rehabilitation.

He was joined by Pvts. Warren Jernegan and Levi Folk of the Hospital Corps.[49] The men believed yellow fever was transmitted by exactly the kind of fomites they were exposing themselves to, and it took real bravery to participate. When the first three volunteers failed to get yellow fever, Reed repeated the experiment two more times with the same results. Traditional sanitation was clearly irrelevant in preventing yellow fever. Two and a half centuries of quarantine and cleaning had been futile. Ultimately Cooke and six enlisted men from the Hospital Corps participated in the experiments. Folk, Jernegan, and James Hanberry volunteered for later experiments and caught yellow fever. That was important as it proved they were not immune during the infected clothing experiments.

At the same time Reed set out to prove the mosquito transmission theory, and in so doing established a standard for medical research that is still followed. First he repeated what Carroll and Lazear had done but with rigid control. The first experimental case of yellow fever at Camp Lazear was in Pvt. John Kissinger, a twenty-three-year-old Ohioan from the Hospital Corps. On November 20 Kissinger was bitten by three infected mosquitoes and bitten again by the same insects three days later. On December 5, he was bitten by five mosquitoes, two of which had fed on patients who later died from yellow fever. On December 9 Kissinger became acutely ill.

Kissinger's roommate, Irishman John J. Moran, served in the VII Corps and the Hospital Corps before resigning to become a civilian clerk on Maj. General Fitzhugh Lee's staff. Moran wanted to go to medical school, and he was convinced the $500 fee being discussed would go a long way toward paying for that. He later thought it over and said if he died he did not want his tombstone to read "Here lie the remains of Johnny Moran, who lost his life in a good cause and spoiled it through accepting AN INSIGNIFICANT REWARD OF $500."[50] He and Kissinger refused to be paid, but they were allowed to choose who they wanted as a doctor and nurse should they get sick. Kissinger was later given a gold watch for his service. As with Folk and Jernegan, Moran participated in later experiments and caught yellow fever.

Between December 5 and February 7, 1901, twelve non-immunes were quarantined and bitten by mosquitoes fed on yellow fever patients. Ten of them got the disease including the two who had been in the infected clothing experiments. Reed said,

> It can readily be imagined that the concurrence of 4 cases of yellow fever in our small command of 12 non-immunes within the space of 1 week, while giving rise to feelings of exultation in the hearts of the experimenters, in view of the vast importance attaching to these results, might inspire quite other sentiments in the bosoms of those who had previously consented to submit themselves to the mosquito's bite. In fact, several of our good-natured Spanish friends who had jokingly compared our mosquitoes to "the little flies that buzzed harmlessly about their tables" suddenly appeared to lose all interest in the progress of science, and, forgetting for the moment even their own personal aggrandizement intentionally severed their connection with Camp Lazear. Personally, while lamenting to some extent their departure, I could not but feel that in placing themselves beyond our control they were exercising the soundest judgement.[51]

Agramonte was more sanguine: "Our artificial epidemic of yellow fever was temporarily suspended while a new batch of susceptible material was brought in, observed, and selected."[52] By December 30, the experiments were back on track and the participants in the fomite study, realizing that they were at no risk, breathed a sigh of relief.

All the yellow fever cases at Camp Lazear were the direct result of experimental inoculation. Of fourteen total cases at the camp none died. In that Reed was remarkably lucky. Any questions about the Carroll, Lazear, and Dean cases had been put to rest. Reed wrote his wife,

Rejoice with me, sweetheart, as aside from the antitoxin of Diphtheria and Koch's discovery of the tubercle bacillus, it will be regarded as the most important piece of work scientifically, during the 19th Century. I do not exaggerate, and I could shout for very joy that Heaven has permitted me to establish this wonderful way of propagating Yellow fever. It was Finlay's theory and he deserves much credit for having suggested it, but as he did nothing to prove it, it was rejected by all, including Genl. Sternberg. Now we have put it beyond Cavil. It's [*sic*] importance to Cuba and the United States cannot be estimated. Major Kean says that the discovery is worth more than the cost of the Spanish War including lives lost and money expended.[53]

The *Stegomyia* theory of transmission was proven, but there were several questions still to answer.

The best scientific experiments create a situation in which everything is held constant except one variable, and that is exactly what Reed did. He constructed another tightly built hut eighty yards across a narrow ravine from Building No. 1. It was of similar size but divided in half by a floor-to-ceiling screen. Entry was through a vestibule similar to Building No. 1 but built to keep mosquitoes in rather than out. The only furniture was a cot with steam-sterilized bedding pushed against each side of the screen. A small laboratory where mosquitoes were bred was attached to the building.[54] Subjects were on both sides of the screen, but mosquitoes that fed on yellow fever victims were introduced to one side only. They were the sole variable. The inoculation volunteers were kept in the hut long enough to be bitten several times—usually about twenty minutes—and then removed to quarantine tents. The controls slept on the other side for up to eighteen nights.

On December 21, Moran stripped, laid on the cot, and allowed himself to be bitten by fifteen mosquitoes during three sessions while Reed watched from the other side of the screen. He contracted what Reed called " a very pretty case" of yellow fever that lasted ten days. When Moran showed Reed his fever chart, "I venture to say that the smile of satisfaction on his face could not have been broader had he been notified by the Secretary of War of his promotion to the rank of Colonel." Reed said, "Moran this is one of the happiest days of my life."[55] Moran spent his ten days on a diet of cracked ice, melon juice, sips of champagne, and ice-water enemas. He said, "The pains I suffered on Christmas night were too intense for description. . . . So it was for the next three days when my pains began to disappear, but I was almost wild for want of sleep. . . . I came out minus about twenty pounds of flesh, and do not care for any more yellow fever. . . . I wish that those who are inclined to disbelieve that mosquitoes are capable of conveying yellow fever would try them just once."[56]

Reed presented the findings at the Pan-American Medical Congress in Havana on February 6, 1901, and published them as "The Etiology of Yellow Fever—An Additional Note" in the *Journal of the American Medical Association*. He returned to Washington in March and never went back to Cuba. He had proven (1) *Stegomyia* (later *Aedes*) was the intermediate host for yellow fever, (2) yellow fever is transmitted by a mosquito feeding on a patient with the disease and biting a non-immune individual, (3) twelve days elapse between the time a mosquito feeds on a yellow fever patient and can transmit the disease, (4) yellow fever is not transmitted by fomites, (5) the only way a building is infectious is if a contaminated mosquito is present, (6) yellow fever spread can be controlled by controlling mosquitoes and keeping them away from sick individuals, and, parenthetically, (7) the specific germ causing yellow fever remained to be identified.

Shortly after returning to Washington Reed became embroiled in a bitter dispute with Sternberg over credit for the commission's work. Sternberg wrote, "Having for years given thought to this subject, I became some time since impressed with the view that in yellow fever as in malarial fevers there is an 'intermediate host.' I therefore suggested to Dr. Reed, president of the board appointed on my recommendation for the study of this disease to the Island of Cuba, that he should give special attention to the possibility of transmission by some insect. . . . I also urged that efforts should be made to ascertain definitely whether the disease can be communicated from man to man by blood inoculations."[57] Reed expressed his concern about priority to Kean who assured him Wood would keep him "perfectly safe from all attempts to rob you of any part of your credit."[58]

Sternberg's one accurate claim was that he encouraged blood inoculation experiments. Those experiments started on January 4 when Walter Jernegan, who had been in both Buildings No. 1 and 2 without catching yellow fever, was injected with two ccs of blood from a Spanish volunteer who had gotten yellow fever from a "loaded" mosquito. He got yellow fever, and 1.5 cc of his blood was injected into William Olsen who got the disease as well. On January 22, 0.5 cc of blood from a severe yellow fever case was injected into Wallace Forbes who also got the disease. A planned fourth experiment was aborted when the volunteer backed out. Reed offered to take his place, but John Andrus, a twenty-one-year-old private in the Hospital Corps who worked in Reed's laboratory, offered to do it instead. The offer was accepted with conspicuous haste, and Andrus was injected on January 25. "The doctor scrubbed a spot on my arm with a piece of alcohol-saturated cotton, inserted a hypodermic needle, slowly pressed the plunger and I was richer by one cubic centimeter of blood taken but a moment before from a vein of a fellow-soldier, Wallace Forbes. At that time his temperature was 102.6°F and he was at the height of a pronounced case of yellow fever."[59]

Wood was fully aware of the risks his soldiers were taking. He wrote Sternberg that Andrus "seems to have acquired a very serious infection. . . . Should he die I shall regret that I ever undertook this work."[60] But the experiment proved beyond question that the yellow fever germ was in the blood and could be transmitted from patient to patient.

There were still questions to answer, two of which required additional mosquito bite experiments. The first was how long the germ had to live in the mosquito before it could be transmitted. To do that volunteers were bitten by the same "loaded" mosquito five days after it fed on a yellow fever patient and then every five days thereafter. The average external incubation period was, as predicted, between eleven and fourteen days.

The second was how long after "loading" the mosquitoes remained capable of transmitting the disease. That would be key to any eradication program. Mosquitoes were fed on a patient in his third day of yellow fever and fed only sugar water thereafter. At thirty-nine days they were allowed to bite Folk who got the disease. Six days later they were allowed to bite Edward Weatherwalks who had participated in the contaminated building experiment. He never became ill and may have been immune. Clyde West, a private in the Eighth Infantry, was bitten on day fifty-one and got yellow fever. James Hanberry, another Hospital Corps member and veteran of Building No. 1, was bitten on day fifty-seven and got the disease. Plans to extend the experiment failed when the sixty-five-day volunteer backed out and mosquitoes intended for days sixty-nine and seventy-one died. Still the commission proved that infected mosquitoes were capable of transmitting yellow fever for at least eight weeks.

The etiological agent remained to be identified. Welch reached out to Reed with work done by Germans Friedrich Löeffler and Paul Frosch who had run plasma through a Berkefeld filter small enough to remove all bacteria. The filtered plasma was still able to transmit the highly infectious cattle hoof and mouth disease, proving the presence of an ultramicroscopic organism, a possibility suggested by Sternberg years earlier. Carroll returned to Havana in August, borrowed infectious mosquitoes, and infected a volunteer. He took plasma from that patient after yellow fever developed, filtered it, and injected the fluid into three volunteers. They got yellow fever, and the circle was closed. Yellow fever was caused by a germ smaller than bacteria that was incubated in and transmitted by the *Stegomyia* mosquito. The Army Board had produced twenty-two cases of yellow fever, sixteen from mosquitoes (eighteen if Lazear and Carroll are counted), and six from injections. Lazear was the only fatality. Volunteer experimental subjects included four army surgeons, two American civilians, ten members of the hospital corps, one soldier, and seven Spaniards and Cubans.

In twenty-five months the Commission comprised entirely of Army surgeons had definitively characterized a disease that had killed tens of thousands over two and a half centuries.

The Army had not waited for the final results. On October 13, 1900, Kean informed his adjutant general that

1. Mosquitoes had been established as the mode of transmission of yellow fever.
2. Mosquito bars (nets) should be placed in all barracks and hospitals.

3. Post commanders should control the mosquitoes by coating the surface of all standing water with petroleum. An ounce of kerosene should be spread over every fifteen square feet including water buckets, fire buckets, undrained puddles, post holes, etc., once a month.[61]

A week later Maj. Gen. Fitzhugh Lee, commander of VII Corps, issued the instructions without change as Circular No. 8. In December the order was extended to every military installation on the island.

Yellow fever patients were treated in screened cages to keep mosquitoes from feeding on them and spreading the disease. Buildings in which yellow fever cases had occurred were fumigated with sulfur or formaldehyde. Pyrethrum insect powder was distributed. Standing fresh water was drained, covered, or oiled. Yellow fever on a base was treated as a command failure.

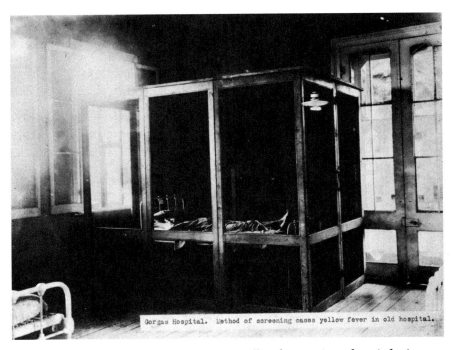

Screened hospital beds were used to prevent yellow fever patients from infecting others. *National Library of Medicine*

Maj. William Gorgas, chief sanitary officer of Havana, remained a mosquito skeptic. After Reed's experiments he reluctantly admitted that mosquitoes might transmit yellow fever but still held that it was not the most common method, and he did not start mosquito control in the city until March 1901. Gorgas was still disinfecting bedding and clothing six months after Reed proved it was unnecessary.

When mosquito control finally started "kerosene squads" were deployed to coat pools, and a few thousand homeowners with standing water on their property were issued $5 fines. In March 1901, there were about 26,000 water supplies with mosquito larvae in Havana. The following January there were fewer than three hundred.

And this time sanitation worked. In January 1901, there were seven yellow fever cases in Havana; in February there were five; in March, one. And there were none in April, May, and June and none from September 1901 to July 1902. Between 1853 and 1900, Havana lost 35,952 people to yellow fever, and it had been 150 years since the city had three straight months without a single case.

What followed was the ultimate irony. Gulf Coast American cities had spent huge amounts of money over the years quarantining ships from Havana in fever season. When the disease broke out in New Orleans in 1905, Havana instituted its own quarantine—on ships arriving from the United States.

PHYSICIANS AND THEIR SUBJECTS

It is worth a moment on what became of some of the participants. In 1929, Congress listed a roll of honor and awarded each a gold medal and a pension. The enlisted participants left the Army anywhere from a few months to twenty-five years after the Cuban experiments, and little is known of their later lives except for a few. William Dean left the service and returned home. Congress subsequently granted Dean a $12-a-month pension, which increased to $125 in 1929. John Kissinger left the service partially disabled from his yellow fever, and his wife was forced to take in laundry to support them. John Moran started medical school at the University of Virginia, but he ran out of funds and went to Panama to work with Gorgas. He later worked in Venezuela, Mexico City, and Havana and served as a

U.S. Army captain in World War I. Forbes had a chronic desertion problem. He repeatedly disappeared and reappeared until 1926 when he went missing and did not return. General Douglas MacArthur said he would be treated as a hero rather than as a deserter if he came back. He did not. James Hanberry was the last survivor; he died in the Veterans Administration Hospital in Columbia, South Carolina, in 1961.

Carlos Finlay was named director of sanitation in the Ministry of Health of the Republic of Cuba in 1902 and held that post until retiring. By that time he had been first author of 264 papers and had been nominated for the Nobel Prize in Physiology or Medicine by both Ronald Ross and Charles Laveran but never received the award. He died at age eighty-two in Havana on August 20, 1915.

William Gorgas took charge of sanitation during construction of the Panama Canal and was named surgeon general in 1914. An annoyed Kean remarked, "So Gorgas got the reward, as was the rule of the Fates that Reed should sow and Gorgas should reap the harvest."[62] He took ill in London where he had gone to receive an honorary knighthood from King George V. The king bestowed the award in the hospital shortly before Gorgas died.

Leonard Wood went on to become the commanding general of U.S. Army forces in the Philippines and commanding general of the Army. To his great disappointment he was passed over for command of the American Expeditionary Force in World War I and did not serve in France. He was the leading candidate for the Republican nomination for president until Warren G. Harding snatched that nomination away in the "smoke-filled room" convention in Chicago in 1920. Wood died from surgery performed by Harvey Cushing to remove a benign brain tumor in 1927.

Jefferson Kean stayed with Wood in Havana until 1906 when he became assistant to the surgeon general. During World War I he served as director of the American ambulance service and rose to the rank of brigadier general. He also founded the Monticello Association of Thomas Jefferson's descendants and consulted on the design of the Jefferson Memorial before his death in 1950.

Lazear, of course, died in Cuba. His supporters campaigned for years for a pension for his widow, which congressional committees denied as setting a troublesome precedent.

Aristides Agramonte earned a second medical degree from the University of Havana in 1900 and took the chair in bacteriology and experimental pathology at that institution. He later became professor of tropical medicine at Louisiana State University School of Medicine and died in 1931.

James Carroll finally received a commission as lieutenant in the Medical Corps in 1902. He succeeded Reed as curator of the Army Medical Museum and wrote the chapter on yellow fever in Osler's *Practice of Medicine*. In later life he harbored intense resentment of Reed's having gotten the lion's share of credit for the yellow fever experiments. He died on September 16, 1907.

After leaving Cuba in 1901, Reed never returned. He went back to being the curator of the Army Medical Museum and taught bacteriology and clinical microscopy at the Army Medical School and pathology and bacteriology at Columbian. He published two later papers on yellow fever before dying of a ruptured appendix on November 23, 1902.[63]

The yellow fever virus was finally isolated by Adrian Stokes in 1927. Max Theiler ran the organism through almost two hundred passages in culture to develop a weakened strain that could be used as a vaccine. Theiler received the Nobel Prize in Physiology or Medicine in 1951, the only Nobel awarded for yellow fever work. His vaccine included 10 percent dilution with human serum to make it easier to filter. Unfortunately, the serum in some lots was contaminated with unrecognized hepatitis virus that caused a serious outbreak of that disease in World War II among American troops vaccinated for yellow fever.

How did this handful of Army surgeons and twenty-five mostly military volunteers manage to do in two years what the best microbiologists in the world had failed to do in a century? First they had a good hypothetical basis from which to work. Carlos Finlay had made an inspired guess, but he had been unable to prove it without knowing the virus's requisite incubation period in the mosquito. Lazear and Agramonte realized that how yellow fever was transmitted was more important than knowing the etiologic agent. Reed designed a brilliant series of experiments that proved the mosquito theory beyond question. Wood put his reputation on the line to give Reed permission and resources to carry out those experiments. Kean put that information to work before most of his colleagues believed it and paved the way for a new kind of sanitation—Gorgas' mosquito control program that eliminated yellow fever from Havana and set the stage for the triumph in the Canal Zone. Finally Reed's experiments were successful because they were challenge trials in which experimental subjects were intentionally given a potentially lethal disease for which there was no effective treatment. Had they waited to collect data from randomly occurring yellow fever, the results would have taken years instead of months and may not have come at all. The ethics of those experiments are debatable, but their effectiveness and the courage of the young experimental subjects were not.

CHAPTER 4

QUARANTINE

Influenza and the American
Expeditionary Force

THE SETTING

We have recently become distressingly familiar with attempts to control a viral pandemic that are not as effective as we might wish. In the early months of the COVID-19 outbreak there was no vaccine, and the only drug therapies were speculative and ineffective. Even revolutionary vaccines and newly developed therapies ameliorated the epidemic but did not stop it. Initial efforts at control relied almost entirely on quarantine—closing borders, restricting travel, and isolating the infected. The Chinese government boasted of the phenomenal success of draconian quarantine measures, but even after putting more than 370 million people in quarantine, the country was forced to lock down large cities to counter resurgent outbreaks. In the United States, schools and businesses were closed, and mask mandates came and went and came again. Historically quarantine has had little success controlling a virulent airborne virus. Such was the case in 1918, and that failure was multiplied many times over by the exigencies of war.

The United States came late to World War I, but the outcome was still very much in doubt when war was declared in April 1917. Russia was reeling militarily, and in November (October by the Russian calendar) the Bolsheviks seized power and started peace negotiations that ended with the

Treaty of Brest-Litovsk in March 1918. Russia's military collapse allowed Germany to shift manpower to the western front for what its military leaders expected to be a war-winning offensive against exhausted British and French armies. American manpower was critical to counter the impending German offensive. The rush to deploy men and materiel precipitated a pandemic that killed far more people than the war itself.

The weapons deployed to fight influenza in 1918 were profoundly ineffective. Immunization had ameliorated the threat of smallpox for Washington's troops in the American Revolution, but there was no vaccine against influenza. There was no drug to prevent or treat the disease. American military surgeons and administrators had identified the mosquito that carried yellow fever and eliminated them and the disease they carried, but influenza's only vector was infected humans. Sanitation had failed for lack of use in nineteenth-century typhoid. Military surgeons were determined not to repeat those errors in 1917, but measures that worked against typhoid did nothing to stop airborne transmission of the influenza virus. Quarantine was always the least of the weapons and was virtually impossible in wartime. In fact troop movements—the diametric opposite of quarantine—in 1918 precipitated the greatest pandemic in history.

The influenza pandemic profoundly affected the war effort and humbled military surgeons accustomed to a string of recent victories over infectious diseases. To understand what happened we need to know something about the pathogen, the situation, and the reaction to what became a pandemic catastrophe.

THE VIRUS

The influenza virus is smaller and less complicated than either pox virus or flaviviruses, and its biology, although complicated, has been well worked out. Influenza is an RNA virus of the *Orthomyxoviridae* family, which has three subtypes based on which nucleoprotein (NP) is present—A, B, or C. Only A and B cause human disease, and only A causes epidemics. The virion is either an irregular sphere or a three-hundred-nanometer filament, both of which have spikes of hemagglutinin (HA) and neuraminidase (NA) protruding from a lipid outer coat. Inside the envelope is a single helical strand of RNA composed of eight chromosomes that encode the virus's ten protein components. Two of the viral proteins (NS1 and NS2 or NEP) are nonstructural. NS1 provides the virus with some protection from interferon, and NS2 helps move viral components between the host nucleus and cytoplasm. PA, PB1, and PB2 are involved in transcribing RNA and producing new viral components. NP surrounds the viral RNA and M2 forms the inner layer of the final virus particle. M1 forms a matrix around the viral core. That is eight and leaves the two proteins that are the most epidemiologically interesting, hemagglutinin and neuraminidase (HA and NA).

The HA spike is lollipop shape with a bulb designed to cling to the sialic (N-acetylneuraminic) acid receptors that are abundant on the surface of respiratory tract epithelial cells. Each bulb has five amino acids that participate in the attachment. Once hooked on the outside of the host epithelial cell the virus is swallowed up and brought into the host cell cytoplasm where the RNA core is uncoated. The viral components then migrate into the host cell nucleus where transcriptase proteins turn the RNA into a messenger RNA (mRNA) that goes back out to the host cytoplasm to direct production of new viral components. Viral RNA (vRNA) is left behind to be the genetic core of a new virus. The interior proteins (NP, M1, PA, PB1, and PB2) are manufactured in the host cytoplasm and return to the nucleus for reassembly with the vRNA. The HA, NA, and M2 migrate to the surface of the host cell and attach to the cell membrane. When the core of the new virion is complete it migrates out of the nucleus and to the surface where it picks up a section of host cell membrane containing M2 and studded with about five hundred HA and one hundred NA molecules. The NS2 breaks the connection between HA and the host's sialic acid receptors, and the new virus is free to bud out and seek a new host.

Influenza has an ecological niche in the intestines of waterfowl, especially ducks and gulls, that allows the virus to travel stunning distances. Migratory birds winter in the tropics, but in the summer the birds congregate in the Arctic where those from Asia and the Americas mix and share viruses.

Influenza also infects a variety of mammals including horses, bats, seals, and pigs. The last is particularly important because swine are capable of hosting both human and avian versions of the virus. Most influenza strains do not cross readily from one mammalian species to another, but pigs and humans are an exception. An avian virus that is not harmful to humans may infect a pig where it can pick up proteins from a version that does infect humans and produce a new pathogen. An infection that is mild or asymptomatic in pigs may be devastating if it crosses over to a human, and human viruses can go back to be harbored in pigs where they may or may not be symptomatic but can share proteins with the pig virus and make new infectious variants.

There are currently eighteen known types of HA and eleven types of NA that can come together in any combination, although not all combinations cause human disease. Once a host has encountered a specific combination—H2N2 for instance—immunity will protect the host from further infection by that combination, but the immunity is not complete. Minor changes in the amino acids on the HA surface can impair immunity and make the virus more infectious, more virulent, or both. These alterations—antigenic drift—account for most of the seasonal variation in influenza types.

A host can be infected by more than one influenza virus at a time, and a real threat arises when the RNA segments from two virions mix or reassort. It is, for instance, possible that a human influenza virus with an HA to which people have become immune reassorts and picks up an avian HA that humans have never encountered. The new virus circumvents immune memory and can infect without impediment. This "antigenic shift" to a new pathogen is what causes pandemics, and that is almost certainly what happened sometime between 1900 and 1918.

We know a good deal about what occurred thanks to three victims of the 1918 pandemic. U.S. Army Pvt. Roscoe Vaughan died of influenza at Camp Jackson outside Columbia, South Carolina. Pvt. James Downs died at Camp Upton sixty-five miles east of New York City on Long Island. Both were subsequently autopsied, and specimens were preserved in the Army Medical Museum (now the Armed Forces Institute of Pathology). A third specimen was disinterred from the grave of a woman who died at Brevig Mission on Alaska's Seward Peninsula and was buried in the permafrost. All three yielded enough tissue to allow sequencing of the virus responsible for the lethal fall wave of influenza. It was H1N1.

There is reasonable evidence that a human virus that emerged some-time before 1907 with human H1 acquired avian N1 neuraminidase and internal protein genes effectively creating a virus to which no one was immune. The lethal variant eventually reassorted and quietly vanished from humans around 1922, but it took refuge in swine where it lived on waiting to be discovered by virologists almost a century later.[1]

Reassortment is not the only way RNA viruses evade the immune system. When the negative sense viral RNA is transcribed to mRNA mistakes are made. Transcription in DNA organisms is not such a serious problem because those organisms come with proofreading mechanisms that destroy faulty copies. That proofreading is not present in RNA viruses, so transcription errors are common, and each error is capable of making a "new" organism; and viral reproduction is awesomely fast. It takes a human around twenty-five years to make a new copy of itself. An influenza virus can do that 10,000 times in six hours with a mutation rate a million times that of a cellular organism.

Hosts defend themselves from viruses in several ways. Most mammals produce chemicals that attack pathogens, the best known of which is interferon. These chemicals are independent of the cellular immune system, but if a host has previously encountered a pathogen he or she can rapidly produce "neutralizing antibodies" that recognize parts of the five amino acids on the HA bulb and bind to them so the virus cannot attach to that host's sialic acid receptors. Hosts with prior exposure can also produce T lymphocytes that kill an infected host cell before viral replication can be completed.

INFLUENZA IN HISTORY

All that helps explain the worst pandemic in human history—at least the worst so far. Influenza or something like it has been around for at least two and a half millennia. Thucydides and Hippocrates described epidemics with symptoms very like modern influenza that struck Athens in 431 BCE and again in 412 BCE. Influenza probably hampered the Roman siege of Syracuse in 212 BCE. An epidemic apparently spread by traveling churchmen swept through England in 664 CE, and Charlemagne's army suffered from "febris italicus" in 876. England and the rest of Europe were swept with an "inflammatory plague" in 1173–74, and an epidemic in Florence in 1357 brought the first clinical use of the term from *influenza di freddo*. Columbus probably brought influenza to the New World in 1493.

The first well-documented influenza epidemic cost Mary I of England 6 percent of her subjects in 1557, and a true pandemic swept across Europe, the Americas, and Africa in 1580. After that pandemics were a regular occurrence (1658, 1679, 1708, 1729–33, 1768, 1781, 1788–90, 1830–33, 1836–37, 1847–50). In 1889 a pandemic (possibly H2N8) that started in Russia killed more than 1 million people and may have infected 40 percent of the world's population. A probable H3N8 variant that emerged in 1900 was widespread, but it caused less severe disease.[2] After 1918–19, influenza epidemics or threats occurred in 1957, 1968, and 1977. The last was, like 1918, an H1N1 variant and likely originated from a laboratory accident in the Soviet Union.[3]

1918 INFLUENZA—THE FIRST WAVE

The 1918 pandemic was of a different order of magnitude. It is estimated that one-third of the world's population had clinically evident infection (about 500 million people), and as many as 100 million died. The case fatality rate was roughly twenty-five times that of previous influenza pandemics.[4] To understand the effect of the first wave on the war, we need to look briefly at the situation on the western front that summer.

On August 4, 1914, German forces launched an invasion of northern France through Belgium and Luxembourg and advanced to within nineteen miles of Paris before the French Army stopped the juggernaut in the First Battle of the Marne (September 6–12). After British and French forces failed to outflank the Germans they established a defensive line in France that extended from the North Sea and western Belgium to the Swiss border. The British took responsibility for the northern portion of the western front while the French held the part in Lorraine along the Aisne River and the Vosges Mountains.

A stalemate of sorts ensued when repeated Allied offensives to dislodge the invaders failed. The Germans, who were also fighting the Russian Army on the Eastern Front, were content to remain on the defensive in hopes of breaking Allied will (the German offensive at Verdun being a notable exception).

The casualty figures on the western front were staggering with the fighting for Verdun and the British Somme Offensive of 1916 the two most sanguinary episodes. A French offensive in 1917 failed and led to widespread mutinies in the French Army. That same year a final Russian effort against the Germans and Austro-Hungarians also failed with similar consequences for the Russian Army. War weariness played a major role in the Bolshevik seizure of power that fall, and Bolshevik leader Vladimir Lenin took Russia out of the war. Also that fall Italy, which had entered the war on the Allied side in 1915, suffered a near-disastrous defeat in the Battle of Caporetto at the hands of Austro-Hungarian and German forces. Austria-Hungary, however, was also reeling with its leaders trying to leave the war, and war weariness was testing German resolve as well. For the Central Powers to win the war, Germany had to win on the western front. Germany's leaders staked everything on four offensives in the *Kaiserschlacht* (Kaiser Battle) or Ludendorff Offensive (named for German General der Infanterie Erich Ludendorff).

By the end of December 1917 the British draft and volunteers had produced an army of 1,200,000 on the western front to join 2,600,000 French and French colonials facing 2,500,000 Germans, but the apparent strength was misleading. The British troops were largely inexperienced, and France had run out of men to draft. At the same time the German Army shifted forty-eight divisions from the east. In the spring of 1918, 191 German divisions were facing 178 French and British divisions on the western front. Additional manpower was essential if the entente was to survive, and those men could only come from the United States.

THE ARMY MEDICAL CORPS

To understand what came next, it is necessary to look at the American Army Medical Corps. The bureau was less than two decades from a stellar success against yellow fever in the Spanish-American War and an exhaustive and highly critical evaluation of the war's typhoid epidemic. Experience with infectious diseases had moved the United States and the Medical Corps in particular into the vanguard of international medical science.

The Rockefeller Institute made sera to treat pneumonia, dysentery, and meningitis. The Hygienic Laboratory (later to be the National Institutes of Health) in Washington, D.C., made smallpox vaccines as well as tetanus and diphtheria antitoxins. The Army Medical School had created an effective typhoid vaccine. It seemed that humanity's war against infectious diseases was on the verge of being won, and the Medical Corps had played a major role in that success.

Reward for that success was slow in coming, but it came. Although Congress had allocated $50 million to the military in the Spanish-American War, none of that money went to the Medical Corps. The government was not going to repeat that mistake. Pneumonia had been a problem for troops on the Mexican border in 1916, and measles had repeatedly plagued Army camps. Neither would be allowed to return. The Council of National Defense was more concerned with infection than injury, and the council's medical committee charged with preparing for war was composed largely of infectious disease experts rather than trauma surgeons.

William Welch was head of pathology at Johns Hopkins. Although he rarely published original research, Welch was revered for his ability to find and train physicians, many of whom went on both to do groundbreaking research and to start training programs of their own at medical schools across the country. He was an urbane, portly, goateed bachelor notoriously jealous of his privacy.[5] He kept meticulously abreast of the latest research in microbial disease, had trained many of the men doing that work, and was legendarily unflappable.

William Gorgas, heralded for his triumphs over mosquito-borne disease in Cuba and Panama, had been appointed surgeon general of the Army in 1914. Victor Vaughan was dean of the medical school at the University of Michigan and had, along with Walter Reed and Edward Shakespeare, served on the Typhoid Commission. These men were at the forefront of infection control, but their victories had been in diseases transmitted by insects and contaminated food and water. They had never tried to control an airborne epidemic.

After the United States entered the war and the Army underwent an explosive expansion, Vaughan, Welch, F. F. Russell, and Rufus Cole toured the training camps in the south. They were so sure sanitary measures taken after the Typhoid Commission report were adequate that Welch planned to resign his commission and return to Hopkins as soon as the tour was over. They all agreed the infection problem was solved, and Welch saw no further need for his expertise.

The camps may have been in good shape, but the Medical Corps was not. In early 1917 there were only 833 physicians and 403 nurses in the Army Medical Corps. Counting officers, contract surgeons, nurses, and civilian employees, the entire service numbered only 8,634.[6]

By the end of the war the Medical Corps would grow to 354,796—three times the size of the entire 1917 Army. Where the men and women and the necessary equipment and administrative structure to support the war effort were to come from was not at all clear in 1917. The U.S. Army attempted to alleviate its nursing shortage by starting a training program for aides and practical nurses, but the effort was crippled by objections from nursing organizations that feared dilution of the profession. The alternative was the Army School of Nursing, but that institution only enrolled 221 students, and by 1918 it had yet to graduate a single nurse.[7] The American Red Cross did bring 21,000 women into the nursing service, but they got them from civilian hospitals that were left starved for staff.

The Hospital Corps grew from 7,000 to 281,000 personnel, and Medical Department hospitals grew from 9,500 beds to 120,900.[8] As with nurses the wartime expansion robbed the civilian healthcare system of its most productive physicians. Half of the physically fit doctors under age forty-five enlisted, leaving mostly physically impaired physicians and those trained before the revolutionary change in American medical education to care for the civilian population.

INFLUENZA IN THE CAMPS

Camp Funston was the beginning. The facility occupied two thousand acres of the Fort Riley reservation near Junction City, Kansas. It was the largest of the sixteen cantonments built during the war and was far from the most pleasant. Captain Francis Blake wrote: "No letter from my beloved for two days, no cool days, no cool nights, no drinks, no movies, no dances, no club, no pretty women, no shower bath, no poker, no people, no fun, no joy, no nothing save heat and blistering sun and scorching wind and working all hours and lonesomeness and general hell—that's Fort Riley, Kansas."[9] It was so hot at Camp Riley that bacteriologists put their cultures in incubators to keep them cool.

The camp was constructed beginning in July 1917, and it grew to 4,000 buildings housing 40,000 troops most of whom would comprise the 89th Infantry Division. The two-story barracks were 140-by-43-foot structures with 150-bed sleeping rooms on each floor. In addition to the barracks the camp had mess halls, assembly halls, schools, libraries, and theaters, all of which were crowded. The men came in trains crammed elbow to elbow. Urban and rural, farm and city boys with entirely separate exposure to infectious diseases were packed in dangerously close quarters.[10]

Fort Riley was also in the heart of the agricultural Middle West. Counties around the fort had upwards of 34,000 hogs, and this may have had something to do with the sudden outbreak of influenza in Haskell County in 1918. Haskell, about three hundred miles east of Camp Funston, was one of the poorest counties in Kansas and was mostly populated by sod house farmers raising pigs and poultry and corn. The Haskell Institute—a school for Indians at Lawrence—was its largest business.

The *Public Health Report* of March 30 included a report from Haskell physician Loring Minor of eighteen cases of influenza with three deaths that had occurred the prior January. The report is odd in that influenza was not a reportable disease, but the Kansas doctor thought the outbreak so unusual that he reported it to the Public Health Service anyway. In February three men from Haskell (Dean Nilson, Ernest Elliot, and John Bolton) visited Camp Funston. The morning of March 4 mess cook Albert Gitchell reported to the camp's infirmary with headache, sore throat, and fever. By lunchtime one hundred more men with similar symptoms had come in, and within weeks a hangar had been converted into a makeshift hospital to handle the flood of patients.[11] Then influenza appeared in cities throughout the Midwest.

After a one-to-five-day incubation period first wave influenza erupted so suddenly that most victims could remember the exact hour they got sick. "The disease began with absolute exhaustion and chill, fever, headache, conjunctivitis, pain in the back and limbs, flushing of face. . . . Coughing was often constant. Upper air passages were clogged."[12] Those symptoms almost certainly coincided with viral invasion of the lining cells of the respiratory tract. The patient's temperature hovered around 100°F. Occasionally there were symptoms of more generalized viral infection including muscle aches, dizziness, insomnia, and loss of the sense of smell and taste. One odd side effect was loss of color vision leaving the victim's world gray and flat. All these tended to be transitory, and recovery after seventy-two hours led to the spring influenza being ubiquitously referred to as the "three-day grippe." Recovery was unremarkable in 95 percent of patients, and the British medical journal *Lancet* questioned whether a disease of such short duration should even be called influenza.[13] Welch, Vaughan, and Cole reported that influenza was nothing to worry about. Although some Army units saw an incidence as high as 90 percent there were very few deaths, and the seemingly benign illness appeared to have run its course by early summer.[14]

Although influenza patient autopsies from later in 1918 left RNA that could be sequenced and definitively labeled as H1N1, there are no such specimens from the early cases, so it is not possible to be certain where the disease originated. An outbreak of purulent bronchitis beginning in December 1916 and peaking the following January and February had occurred at the British camp in Étaples and at Aldershot across the Channel, but unlike the spring version of influenza elsewhere this was quite virulent with a high mortality from secondary pneumonia. It was suggested that German gas attacks, the filth of the trenches, and overcrowding may have allowed an otherwise mild illness to be lethal, but it seems more likely that this was just not the same disease.[15]

China has also been suggested as an origin of the pandemic. Maintaining the western front required manual laborers, and some 140,000 Chinese arrived in 1917 and 1918. Some of them came through Vancouver and crossed Canada and the United States by train on their way to the ships that would take them across the Atlantic to France. There had been an outbreak of pulmonary disease in China in 1917, and it has been suggested that infected laborers spread influenza while crossing North America. There is, however, no record of any of those workers being ill, and the lethal 1917 and 1918 outbreak in China may have been pneumonic plague anyway.[16]

While the exact origin of the 1918 influenza is uncertain, there is no question that Camp Funston's cases were the first in the U.S. Army and predated the widespread European outbreak by several weeks. The first wave of the pandemic crossed the United States in March, April, and May before tearing through Europe in May, June, and July.

This wave was highly infectious but not especially virulent. It made people sick, but it rarely killed them. Patients were advised to rest and gargle a chlorine solution and sniff warm water every four to six hours, to cover their mouths when coughing, and to wash their hands and burn their handkerchiefs. There was no effective treatment for the disease, but none was needed. It just had to run its course.[17]

Even though it was mild and self-limited, the first wave of influenza had a dramatic effect on the military, first in the American cantonments in the United States and then in the camps and trenches of Europe. The thirty-two large American training camps were designed to wedge 25,000 to 50,000 recruits into claustrophobically small spaces. In the winter months of 1918 even those buildings were incomplete, and many men were housed in tents.

Quarantine was the only weapon against the airborne virus, and in a military preparing for war there was no effective way to segregate the well from the infected. The U.S. Army grew from 378,000 men to 4.7 million, all of whom had to be trained. Physician historian Percy Ashburn wrote: "They were shifted from camp to camp by thousands, taking with them such diseases as they were incubating, thus infecting all camps as impartially as human ingenuity, or lack of it, could assure."[18] Between March and May, fourteen of the training camps suffered outbreaks. The War Department enlisted 158,000 students in 500 colleges in the Student Army Training Corps program virtually assuring the spread of infection on college campuses. When troops were sent to the western front they took influenza with them.

A large-scale movement of American troops began in March with 84,000 men shipped to France and 118,000 more the following month.[19] The first group of new troops landed at Bordeaux in southwestern France in April, and influenza came with them. Although the disease was mild, its effect was not. Influenza swept through France with up to 30 percent

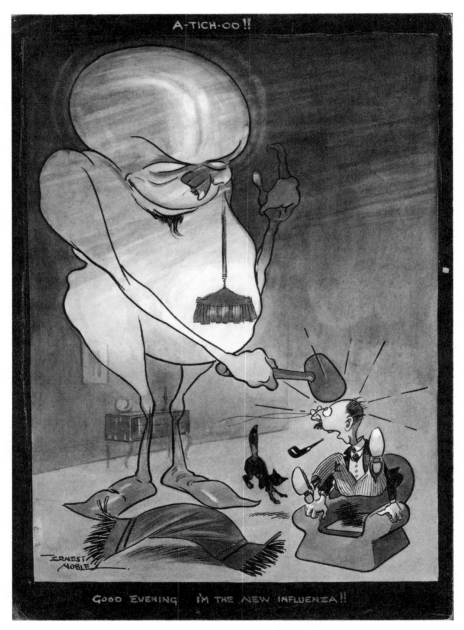

Pen-and-ink drawing by E. Noble, ca. 1918. The influenza "monster" could not be controlled with quarantine or sanitation, and there was neither an effective medication nor a vaccine in 1918. *Wellcome Library*

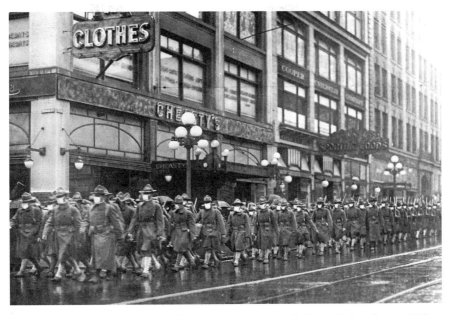

Masked soldiers of the U.S. Army's 39th Regiment march through Seattle, ca. 1918, prior to departing for France during World War I. *NARA*

of affected American units sick. By early June there were cases in the American Expeditionary Force's (AEF) units from the Somme to Lorraine. Replacements were coming in four-thousand-man brigades that moved every three to four weeks. When men in the front line became ill, they were replaced by a fresh supply of men without immunity, and the virus got a flood of new hosts. It is impossible to know exactly how many cases of influenza there were in the AEF since it was not a reportable disease until after June 15, 1918, but if the camps where it was recorded were an indication the numbers were staggering.

The British Expeditionary Force (BEF) kept some numbers, and they were impressive. The epidemic began in the First and Second Armies in April and May and spread to the Third and Fourth Armies, each of which saw 2,000 to 4,000 cases a week. From May 18 to June 2 the First Army reported 36,473 hospitalizations for influenza.[20] Only about 1 percent of those infected got pneumonia, although 10–15 percent of those who did died. These numbers are a bit deceptive since roughly 90 percent of those with influenza were treated at casualty clearing stations or in their own barracks and were never reported. Nonetheless, 200,825 British troops were unable to report for duty in June and July.[21]

The Royal Navy recorded 10,313 cases of influenza in May, and the fleet was unable to put to sea for three weeks even though only four sailors died from the disease.[22] The disease rendered a large proportion of the naval forces temporarily ineffective, but almost everyone who contracted influenza recovered.

The epidemic struck the French Army in early April as well with more than 40,000 troops hospitalized for influenza.[23] That spring three-fourths of French frontline troops reported sick. French soldiers on leave brought the disease to Paris in late April. The same happened in London and the rest of Britain.

The disease appeared in Germany in June, Denmark and Norway in July, and Sweden and the Netherlands in August. Before the year was out it had struck British colonies in Bombay, Calcutta, Madras, and Rangoon.

Sensitive to the possibility that news of a pandemic would adversely affect the war effort, the domestic press in both Europe and the United States played down the disease. The American press minimized what was happening in the camps, saying it was just "la grippe" with the same old fever and chills that accompanied any seasonal illness. Because Spain was not a combatant the Spanish press was far more open about the pandemic's risks and published more detailed accounts. Their reward was to have the disease named Spanish flu.

German Kaiser Wilhelm II initially suggested that the illness among the Allied armies would tilt the war on the western front in Germany's favor, but he was proved disastrously wrong. By late April, "Blitzkatarrh" was racing through his troops. Between March and July 1.75 million German soldiers reported sick in a stretch when only 750,000 were lost to wounds.[24] The numbers went up so quickly that the overwhelmed German doctors just stopped recording them.

Ludendorff had planned a multipronged thrust into the Allied lines north and south of the Somme to separate the French sector from the British. He reasoned that if he could defeat the demoralized French Army and push the British forces up against the Channel the British would withdraw from the war. He thought he would be most successful north of the

Somme, but when he launched the attack on March 2 it was south of the river that his thrust was successful. There Ludendorff's troops advanced some forty miles, took 80,000 prisoners, captured 975 artillery pieces, and cut the main rail line to Paris.

Then he stopped. Historian Basil Liddell Hart attributed this to fear of an Allied counterattack, but Ludendorff had 208 divisions and another 80 in reserve and the Allies were in no shape to take the offensive. In his July 7, 1918, diary entry, Army surgeon Harvey Cushing wrote: "Wonderful weather continues and yet no renewal of Boche offensive. Many theories— shortage of men? Internal troubles? An epidemic of the 3-day fever? Preparation for some sort of surprise? Meanwhile he's losing his most valuable ally—time. Our people are coming fast."[25] Later in that entry he concluded, "No one understood why Germans were withdrawing. Something must be happening to the Boches. . . . No equal spectacle of German indecision since the war began."[26]

What Cushing did not know was that the German were suffering far more from influenza than the British and French. It is true the German forces were low on fuel and ammunition and dealing with long supply lines and poor roads, but influenza had devastated the army. Thousand-man battalions were cut in half. Ludendorff wrote: "It was a grievous business having to listen every morning to the Chiefs of Staff's recital of the number of influenza cases, and their complaints about the weakness of their troops."[27]

Ludendorff tried to push forward and take the railroad center at Amiens, but on August 8—the "Black Day" in Germany—forward movement stopped. Cushing summed up: "Certainly something unaccountable has happened to the Boches. They seem to be beating a retreat toward the old Hindenburg Line before the British, who are clinging to their heels. . . . Can it be the Boches have cracked?"

They had. Ludendorff informed his superiors that his ailing army could no longer be relied upon. It was the beginning of the end of the German military effort. The offensive that could have ended the war with a German victory was hampered by long supply lines with shortages of fuel and ammunition, but mostly it fell victim to a virus.[28]

THE SECOND WAVE

On both sides of the front influenza abated in August, and it was generally assumed the epidemic was over. It was not. The virus probably started mutating as early as April, but it was late summer before the change was evident. When influenza returned it came with a vengeance. The new outbreak was so different that many thought it was a different disease altogether. Physicians suggested that something in the war—chemicals from explosives, gas warfare, or a super germ arising from rotting corpses—was responsible.

The best argument against it being a different virus was that those who had the disease in the first wave were at least partially immune to the second. One infantry regiment was widely infected in June before being transferred from Hawaii to Camp Dodge in August. When the second wave broke out at Camp Dodge it infected one-third of the troops stationed there and killed almost 7 percent of them, but the regiment from Hawaii was spared.[29]

Incidence of influenza in the cantonments in the United States was significantly higher than among the AEF troops.[30] Although we do not have sequenced RNA from the spring outbreak to prove it, it is likely that the virus mutated and reemerged in camps crowded with men who lacked immunity before being spread when they were deployed. At any rate the influenza that exploded in the late summer and fall of 1918 was radically different from the "three-day grippe" that preceded it.

The first wave likely started in the United States; the second probably started in Great Britain. Plymouth is about 160 miles north of Brest, France, in almost a straight north-south line across the English Channel. Ships regularly departed Plymouth for Brest as well as going across the Atlantic to North America or south to West Africa. The second wave appeared in Plymouth in August just when HMS *Mantua*, a converted liner built for the Peninsula and Orient Australia run, left for Sierra Leone with 600 passengers, 10,000 pounds of meat, and 365 tons of fresh water. On August 8 influenza broke out on board. Two days later there were 25 cases; by August 13 there were 103. When the ship arrived in Sierra Leone there were 124 cases, 10 of whom ultimately died.[31] The infection spread from the *Mantua* to other Royal Navy ships and to the port in September.[32]

An estimated 3 percent of the population of Sierra Leone died of influenza that month.[33]

The second wave came to Brest on August 22. By September 15, 1,350 men had been hospitalized and 370 had died.[34] Influenza arrived in Boston—possibly on a troop ship returning from Plymouth—on August 27 with three cases reported from Commonwealth Pier. Two days later there were fifty-eight more. At first most of those infected were sent to Chelsea Naval Hospital, but the epidemic did not stay with sailors.[35] Within five days the epidemic was in the community, and Boston City Hospital admitted its first cases. Influenza spread to Navy yards in Philadelphia and Newport News, and the same day the first death was reported among civilians in Boston it struck Camp Devens.

Like Camp Funston in Kansas, Devens was a hurriedly built facility designed to house and train a flood of recruits. The five-thousand-acre camp was on the Boston and Maine Railroad line thirty miles northwest of Boston, and although designed for 35,000 men it had ballooned to 45,000 by the time the camp was fully operational in September. Lucky early arrivals slept in one of the 728 new buildings, but 5,000 who came later were relegated to tents.

The 76th Infantry Division—the first to be trained at Camp Devens—was dispatched to France on July 4. The 12th Infantry Division replaced them, and beginning September 12 suffered an explosion of disease so severe it was initially diagnosed as meningitis. There were 31 admissions on July 12; six days later there were 1,176. A hospital designed to handle a maximum of ninety new patients a day was admitting more than one thousand. Ultimately 14,000 men stationed at Devens got influenza, 757 died, and very few ever made it to France.[36]

Welch, Vaughan, and Cole had just finished their report on the camps and were about to tell the surgeon general that sanitation was well in hand and the men were safe from epidemic disease. Gorgas was in Europe when the three returned to Washington, so they met with Acting Surgeon General Charles Richard who presented them with a rude surprise. "You will proceed immediately to Devens. The Spanish influenza has struck that camp."[37] What they found in Massachusetts shook even the impassive Welch. The two-thousand-bed hospital there had eight thousand patients, and ninety of its three hundred nurses were sick. Barracks, mess halls, and tents overflowed with dying soldiers.

Vaughan described what they found: "I see hundreds of young, stalwart men in the uniform of their country coming into the wards of the hospital in groups of ten or more. They are placed on the cots until every bed is full and yet others crowd in. The faces soon wear a bluish cast; a distressing cough brings up blood stained sputum. In the morning the dead bodies are stacked about the morgue like cord wood."[38]

Cole wrote, "Owing to the rush and the great number of bodies coming into the morgue, they were placed on the floor without any order or system, and we had to step amongst them to get into the room where an autopsy was going on."[39] Welch was stunned. "This must be some new kind of infection or plague."[40] He wired Gorgas that this was an emergency and required rapid expansion of hospital facilities. Worse, he knew preparations for deployment meant men would be moving from one camp to another around the country. It was only a matter of time before the disease spread to all the other cantonments. Welsh recommended immediate suspension of transfers in and out of Devens.

The three experts suggested that all beds and mess tables be separated by screens and that the camp be immediately reduced to ten thousand men with a minimum of fifty square feet of barrack space for each man. They reasoned that modest separation might slow airborne movement of the virus from one host to another, although they knew it would not completely stop the spread. This wave of influenza was formidably infectious, and Vaughan quietly admitted they were helpless against the new plague. Welch, Vaughan, and Cole came to regard the epidemic as the greatest failure of medicine in their lifetimes.

Their recommendations came to nothing; Devens' camp commander ignored them all. The camp stayed overcrowded, and troop movements continued. We will never know if sealing Devens off might have stopped the second wave in the United States but sending infected men out to carry the virus to armies of new hosts certainly aggravated what came next.

In this wave Camp Devens suffered 14,784 cases of influenza, 3,743 of whom got pneumonia. Case numbers rocketed up for eight days, peaked October 12, and began a spontaneous precipitous decline over the next month.[41] The second wave was widespread and lethal, but it was self-limited. It may have abated because such a high percentage of people got sick that the virus ran out of hosts, or the virus may have simply evolved into a form that did not cause such severe disease. Whatever happened to the virus, it was in spite of and not because of anything the military did.

The effect of Fort Devens on the commission was devastating. They had trained at the cusp of modern medicine; Koch and Pasteur had rendered diseases that had been unfathomable mysteries for millennia comprehensible. Researchers and military surgeons had deciphered and found ways to control diseases that had killed millions. They had revolutionized medical education and built a system combining patient care, education, and research. Now they were faced with a pandemic, and none of their new knowledge was of any use. They had no vaccine, no effective treatment, nothing to sanitize, and no vector to remove. These heroes of modern science were impotent, and they knew it. Ashburn got straight to the point: "It is a sad story, that of the respiratory diseases and Medicine sits bowed and humbled when it is told. . . . Medicine knows that it has not reached its goal, that the age-long struggle for the master of infections is only partly won, that bitterness and humiliation must yet be drunk."[42]

The inadequacy was even worse in the military. In 1918, medical officers still functioned as consultants to the line officers with no authority to give orders to anyone outside the medical service. The division surgeon's role was sharply circumscribed. He was "charged under the commanding general, with the general conduct and supervision of the Medical Department."[43] A division surgeon's only authority was over his own people, and even that was subject to change from outside the department.

On September 19, the acting surgeon general wrote commanding Gen. Peyton March asking that any "organization known to be infected" not be sent to Europe. Canada was already quarantining all troops for twenty-eight days prior to embarkation, and Welch suggested at least fourteen days for American troops. Gorgas only asked for a week. March offered pre-embarkation physical exams and a 10 percent decrease in the troop ship passenger loads, but he said quarantine was out of the question. He informed President Woodrow Wilson that any decrease in troop transfers would endanger the western front and boost German morale. March prevailed. Americans were critical to halting any German advance. Not incidentally, Wilson and Secretary of War Newton Baker were convinced that a strong American presence before the war ended would enhance Wilson's influence in the anticipated peace settlement.

Gorgas asked for a special quarantine camp to be established at Funston, but that request was refused as well. Commander of the AEF Gen. John J. Pershing said that the French needed a constant supply of new men if they were to survive, and the Medical Corps was not going to stand in the way. Col. S. M. Kennedy, chief surgeon of the New York port of embarkation, knew influenza was likely in the departing ships but said, "We can't stop this war on account of Spanish or any other kind of influenza."[44] Quarantine, the only tool available to fight the influenza pandemic, was simply incompatible with fighting a war.

Only a day after the second wave broke out at Devens the first case appeared at Camp Upton, the embarkation facility on Long Island. Influenza was at Camp Dix in New Jersey September 18, Camp Kearney in California September 27, Camp Funston (again) and Camp Dodge in Iowa September 29, and Camps Wheeler and Greenleaf in Georgia October 11. Men were being shifted by train from camp to camp, and wherever they went influenza went with them.

Up to 40 percent of the U.S. Navy's personnel contracted influenza in 1918 although the morbidity and mortality were less than that in the Army camps. It was in nine Navy camps in the east within a week and thirteen more in the Midwest and South a week later. Sailors carried the disease, and civilians in cities around their ports were infected as well. Influenza was in New Orleans September 4 and in New London September 12. On September 17 several hundred men were transferred from the Philadelphia Navy Yard to Puget Sound. On arrival eleven men had influenza; eight days later the epidemic appeared in Seattle. The Great Lakes naval training facility is thirty miles north of Chicago; influenza appeared there September 11, and 2,600 men were in the base hospital within a week. The disease was epidemic in Chicago eight days later. The Navy saw 106,000 men hospitalized and lost 5,027 to influenza and pneumonia in the second wave—twice as many died from enemy action in the war.[45]

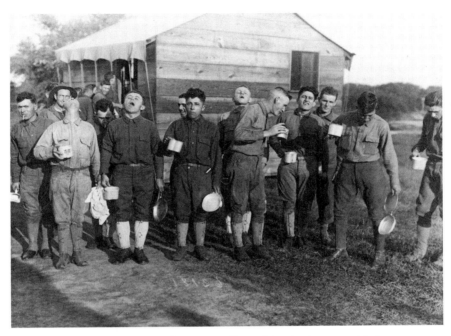

U.S. soldiers at Fort Dix, New Jersey, gargling salt water to prevent influenza, 1918–19. *NARA*

Recruits wanted to get off the bases whenever possible, but local leaders pushed back. On October 19, the Detroit commissioner of health wired commanders of every Midwest training installation that his city was off-limits to all military personnel who did not have a letter from their commanding officer saying they were in perfect health and their travel was absolutely necessary. Camp Funston posted military police at the train station to keep men on base, but there was no consistency in the way camps dealt with the epidemic. Each camp commander held final authority over medical care, and in the absence of national standards, every camp made its own rules.

Some cantonments such as Camp Grant in Illinois did try to protect the well from the infected. "The wearing of masks and gowns, frequent washing of hands and avoiding of putting hands in mouth or nose is very important. Persons must avoid crowding whether on duty or not."[46] Those warnings proved profoundly ineffective. In a single week ten occupied beds in the camp became 4,102, and civilian doctors and nurses had to be brought in from nearby Rockford to handle the flood. Of the camp's 40,000 trainees, 10,713 became sick and 1,060 died.

The only visitors allowed in Camp Grant were relatives who had received "danger or death" telegrams. Even with the restrictions there were so many cases of "danger or death" that the Red Cross had to put chairs and cots in a hastily erected tent to accommodate the deluge. The camp contracted with local undertakers at $50 a body and reassigned any soldiers with embalming experience to handle the overflow. A mortuary built for twelve to fifteen deaths a day had to deal with 117 in mid-October.

Col. Charles Hagadorn, Camp Grant's commanding officer, at first refused to take the outbreak seriously and insisted that his men be housed in regular barracks rather than in isolation tents. On September 20, he moved his men from the tents into crowded buildings over the strenuous objections of his medical staff. The following day influenza came from Camp Devens with a trainload of transfers, and by midnight 108 men had been hospitalized. In six days there were 4,102, and on October 4 more than 100 men died.

Gorgas recommended that all troop movements from the camp be stopped, but he was ignored. On September 28, a train with 3,106 men left Camp Grant for Camp Hancock near Augusta, Georgia. On arrival 700 of them went directly to the hospital. Ultimately 2,000 of the 3,108 transfers were hospitalized, and almost 7 percent of them died.[47]

Inundated with bad news Hagadorn ordered his administrative staff to leave his office building, closed the door, and committed suicide.

In Georgia local undertakers were overwhelmed with bodies from the camps, and embalming supplies had to be brought from as far away as Philadelphia. Camp Greenleaf at Chickamauga National Battlefield Park trained medical units—eventually more than one hundred base, evacuation, and field hospitals—for the AEF. Even the medical training facility was a hotbed of influenza with more than 6,000 cases and 325 deaths.[48]

Some camps increased the amount of space allotted for each man to fifty square feet as recommended by the surgeon general and separated cots with sheets, although there was justifiable skepticism about those measures. Efforts at Camp Humphries in Virginia presaged those that would be used a century later. Medics placed articles on influenza in the camp newspaper: "Influenza is a communicable disease and is transmitted from one person to another through the medium of the fine spray thrown out from the nose or thrown during coughing or spitting. It can be easily controlled. . . . The prevention of disease is simple and consists of avoiding the disgusting habit of coughing in another's face."[49] Noncommissioned officers were posted at entertainment venues to remove anyone coughing without covering his face. Men who coughed in mess halls were forced to leave and were only allowed back after everyone else had eaten. Men were told to bathe at least once a week—twice if possible. But the camp was never quarantined, and the men moved freely around the camp and the surrounding towns.

Something had changed dramatically over the summer. Patients got the usual influenza and seemed to recover, but a distressing number came back one to three weeks later desperately ill with bacterial pneumonia. *Bacillus influenzae* (now *Hemophilus influenzae*) was so common among these patients that it was widely considered the cause of the disease and named accordingly. *Staphylococcus aureus*, *Streptococcus pneumoniae*, and Group A *Streptococcus* were also common.[50] In the absence of antibiotics mortality among the infected was formidable. The sickest patients had acute viral disease and bacterial pneumonia simultaneously. As many as 20 percent of those with the new influenza got pneumonia, and upwards of 37 percent of those died. Fevers of 105°–106°F and delirium were common.

There was one more peculiarity. Ordinary influenza has its highest death rate in the very young and the very old with young adults typically being spared severe illness. In 1918, a majority of the deaths were in twenty-eight to thirty-five-year-olds.[51] The reason for this is somewhat uncertain, but the best guess is that these were the people exposed to H2N8 influenza in 1889–90 or H3N8 in 1900. Those exposed before the earlier pandemics may have come away with an immune system primed for the earlier variants but with an impaired ability to respond to H1N1. That might explain why the death rate in fifteen to thirty-year-olds was twenty times that of prior influenza epidemics, and 99 percent of deaths were in those less than sixty-five years of age. Regardless of the cause the age predilection had obvious military implications.

Disease in the second wave was gruesome. Some patients presented with the sudden onset of what appeared to be destruction of the lining membranes of the entire respiratory tract. Patients coughed up sputum the consistency of tomato purée. "These men start with what appears to be an ordinary attack of La Grippe or Influenza, and when brought to the Hosp. they very rapidly develop the most vicious type of Pneumonia that has ever been seen. Two hours after admission they have the mahogany spots over the cheek bones, and a few hours later you can begin to see the Cyanosis extending from their ears and spreading all over the face, until it is hard to distinguish the coloured men from the white."[52] Patients literally drowned in their own secretions. Men in apparently splendid health and perfect physical condition suddenly became desperately ill, and many of them died in less than forty-eight hours. In one week in October the Medical College of Virginia Unit in France saw over one hundred influenza cases 80 percent of whom died.[53] Pericarditis (inflammation of the cardiac lining), myocarditis (inflammation of the heart muscle), renal failure, and liver failure all occurred. Lungs filled with blood instead of air and took on the consistency of raw liver. Transient cough, fever, and lethargy were followed by rapidly progressive pneumonia with hypoxia and outright respiratory failure. One of the most distressing symptoms was copious epistaxis that occurred in 5–15 percent of cases. It was not just a nosebleed but a hemorrhage that spurted across the room. The patients coughed up a bloody foam, and some bled from the intestines and vomited blood. Nurses had copious menstrual bleeding.

Those who cared for the patients were shocked by the speed with which they deteriorated. "Every one is coughing. Bronchitis is rife and is running a very virulent course. An autopsy showed the bronchi to be filled with pus."[54] Men were more likely to die in the hospital than at the front. "It is only a matter of a few hours until death comes . . . it is horrible. One can stand it to see one, two, or twenty men die. . . . For several days there were no coffins and bodies piled up something fierce. . . . It beats any sight ever had in France after a battle."[55] Lethal pneumonia could start in as little as three to five days and was probably due to virus destroying the lining of the respiratory tract. The raw surface was an ideal site for secondary bacterial infection with *Hemophilus*, *Streptococcus*, or *Staphylococcus*, none of which were treatable in the pre-antibiotic era.

This third version of the disease may have been an unfortunate consequence of an overactive immune system. It is possible that the body's attempt to combat the virus resulted in mass killing of its own cells—a cytokine storm. At any rate this manifestation seems to have been systemic and not the result of direct damage from the virus itself. Regardless, the first wave temporarily sickened large numbers of young people. The second wave killed them.

As bad as things were in the camps, they were worse on the transports taking men to Europe. Camp commanders had reluctantly allowed thirty or even fifty square feet of space per man; troop ships were lucky to have one-fifth of that. Influenza started in the Atlantic ships in late July, earlier than in the camps, and the first cases of pneumonia as a lethal accompaniment to the viral infection were on the ships.

Gens. March and Pershing insisted the Army send as many men to Europe as the ships could carry. March insisted a preboarding physical examination was adequate protection, arguing that if men became sick in transit they could be quarantined in quarters guarded by military police. But those quarters did not exist for troops crammed into four-high flat metal shelves that folded into narrow passageways. Sick men on the fourth level of bunks had the hardest time. They could not get out of the bunk, and overworked caretakers could not get to them. Sleeping quarters reeked. Urine, feces, vomitus, and blood pooled on the decks.

Army nurse Mary Dobson, who got influenza herself on a troop ship, described the experience: "You had terrific pain all over your body, especially back and head, and you just felt as if your head was going to fall off. The odour was terrible in that ship's infirmary—I never smelt anything like it before or since. It was awful because there was poison in this virus."[56]

The SS *Leviathan* was a sad case study. The ship, commissioned as the *Vaterland* in the German merchant fleet, had been seized at Hoboken, New Jersey, when war was declared. It was built to carry 6,800 passengers and crew but had been reconfigured (over the objections of medical officers) to hold 11,000. Under Secretary of the Navy Franklin Roosevelt arrived in New York returning from Brest on the *Leviathan* on September 29 so sick that he had to be taken off the ship on a stretcher and sent directly to the hospital. The ship was moved to Hoboken on October 7 and sent back to France with a fresh load of troops. Influenza broke out within forty-eight hours of sailing, and, by the time she came to Brest, the *Leviathan* had six hundred influenza cases and more than one hundred cases of pneumonia. Sixty-seven men died during the crossing.

A U.S. convoy arrived at St. Nazaire two days ahead of the *Leviathan* with 24,488 men, 4,147 of whom had become sick during the voyage. On reaching port 1,357 were taken to the hospital.[57] In the end it is estimated that over four thousand men died at sea or shortly after their arrival in France in the last two months of the war. The Army started shipping embalming materials with the troops.

The number of sick and dying could not be hidden and became a political liability. President Wilson needed a scapegoat, and Army Commanding General Peyton March was a good candidate. When he was called to the White House March defended himself claiming that the men had been cleared both in the training camps and embarkation ports. Besides the Germans would certainly take comfort if the rate of transport was decreased, and any lives lost to influenza were balanced by those saved in a shorter war. Wilson was convinced. Although the numbers on the transports were reduced so that, by the Armistice, the transports were carrying only 30 percent of their capacity and men were ordered to wear masks on board, the damage had been done.

And the epidemic blazed on. Between September 12 and October 18, there were 274,745 cases of influenza and 46,286 cases of pneumonia with 14,616 deaths in military personnel who never left the United States.[58] There is no glory dying in a hospital before leaving home, and although casualties were publicized in great detail deaths from influenza were not. Gorgas continued to demand that no men be sent to Europe from camps with ongoing influenza outbreaks. March finally and reluctantly agreed, and Provost Marshal Enoch Crowder canceled the 142,000-man October draft because there were no healthy facilities for recruits.

Responsibility for deaths in camps and on ships was a constant source of friction between the Medical Corps and the General Staff. Gorgas went around the military hierarchy to ask Congress for more authority for his medical officers. That infuriated both the War Department and Wilson, and March brought Gorgas in for a dressing down. The situation deteriorated further when *Military Surgeon* editor John R. Van Hoff published an article castigating the War Department for not following medical advice. Secretary of War Newton Baker charged that the editorial showed "a complete disloyalty toward the legally constituted head of the War Department and is calculated to produce friction in the military machine."[59] It cost Van Hoff his job and set the wheels turning toward Gorgas losing his as well.

The usual retirement age for the surgeon general was sixty-four, but Gorgas very much wanted to stay on. Baker sent him on an inspection tour of France as his birthday approached. That is where Gorgas learned from the newspapers that he was to be replaced by Lt. Col. Merritte Ireland.

Influenza among American military personnel in France was not as serious as in the United States and on the ships, but it was bad enough. The supply and rear area units were at more risk than men at the front, and new arrivals remained at risk. Mary Dobson worked on the influenza ward at Savenay because she had the disease on the ship over and was presumed immune. The staff was told there was no influenza in the United States, but they had been at Camp Grant and knew better. Half the patients Dobson worked with came straight off the boat. "They just died within twenty-four hours after they got there. The cemetery was just up the hill and every morning you could hear the bugle blowing as they buried the bodies. It was gruesome. It really was."[60]

Timing of the October outbreak in France could not have been worse. It exactly coincided with Pershing's finally receiving permission for his 1.2 million American troops to operate independently in the Meuse-Argonne in the largest U.S. military action of the war. That month more of Pershing's men were evacuated and hospitalized for influenza than for wounds. Eventually the First Army suffered 93,160 killed and wounded in the Meuse-Argonne Offensive. During the battle, 68,760 men were reported out of action for medical reasons, the vast majority of which were influenza, and that is undoubtedly a serious underestimate since the AEF counted only those cases with a recorded temperature greater than 104°F.

On October 1 Pershing halted the offensive in the face of poor performance by his armies. The fact that there were 16,000 new influenza cases in Pershing's troops the week ending October 5 surely played a part in the poor showing. The pandemic killed more Americans in Europe during the second phase of Meuse-Argonne than in any other month of the war.

Influenza hurt the AEF in several ways. Influenza adversely affected troop morale at the same time loss of officers degraded planning and leadership. The need to evacuate the sick from the front lines used up transportation and clogged the roads. Supplies could not get to the front and men were reduced to foraging for food. Stretcher-bearers were recruited to bring back bread and canned corned beef after dropping off the sick and hurt.[61] Still, the AEF units in France were affected less than personnel in the camps at home. At its peak, hospitalizations in France totaled 167/1,000 men compared to 361/1,000 in the United States.

Problems tend to draw attention when they affect the powerful. Representative Augustus Gardiner of Massachusetts, the first member of Congress to join the Army, died at Camp Wheeler in January, and Congress wanted someone to blame for the ensuing clamor. The Senate Committee on Military Affairs concluded that deaths in the camps were directly attributable to mistakes made by Wilson and the War Department. Victor Vaughan agreed. "Insufficient clothing, overcrowding in tents, barracks and hospitals, and lack of heat in the houses have been potent in the development of pneumonia among our soldiers, and for these deficiencies the medical corps is not responsible."[62] Gorgas told the committee that it was entirely the fault of the General Staff that the men were overcrowded and sick. A January 26 *New York Times* headline read "Gorgas Ascribes Deaths to Haste." Members of the General Staff were furious that Gorgas had gone over their heads to politicians and the press, and they countered that the sickness and death were due to unhealthy recruits and poor medical care and suggested that the doctors be punished for the "incompetence and laxity" in the Medical Corps.

Of course the second wave did not spare the Central Powers. Morale on their side of the front dropped with news of increasing civilian mortality in Germany during October and November. The home front was collapsing, soldiers' families were hungry, and influenza was rampant. Sentries had to be stationed behind the lines to catch men deserting to get back to their families. In five months in 1918 Germany lost 1 million men to injury and disease including some 125,000 dead and 100,000 missing at the same time 1 million American troops were arriving in France.

Austria-Hungary was spared the first wave of influenza, but the empire suffered mightily in October and November of 1918 in the second. It is not a coincidence that the outbreaks in Germany and Austria-Hungary peaked at the same time both governments formally requested armistice negotiations. It did not help that Prince Max of Baden, the new German chancellor, was down with influenza at the same time.

"CONTROLLING" THE EPIDEMIC

From the beginning the usual sanitation measures were ineffective against the epidemic although handwashing and physical separation were encouraged. The Public Health Service advised: "The range of a careless cougher or sneezer is at least 3 feet."[63] There was some civilian evidence that mask mandates and closing schools, churches, and bars prevented disease, but all those measures remained controversial.[64] Quarantine did little or nothing to stop the pandemic, but it was the only thing available.

Available treatments, although numerous, were uniformly useless. A variety of folk remedies including raw onion rubs on the chest, creosote baths, brown sugar, laxatives, and warm foot baths were promoted. Iodine and glycerin mouthwash and mentholated Vaseline in the nose were equally futile. Masks soaked with 1 percent iodine mixed with the nursery cleanser Albolene were ubiquitous on transports and in hospitals but useless as well. Digitalis was given empirically as a cardiac stimulant, but it did more harm than good. Opiates were used to suppress cough but did nothing for the underlying pneumonia.

Vaccination had worked in other diseases and was the siren song of research, but the organism responsible for influenza remained to be identified. Bacteria were considered the likely culprit, and vaccine research was directed against one or another purported pathogen none of which caused the disease. The most popular candidate was the bacillus identified in pneumonia associated with influenza by Richard Pfeiffer, initially referred to eponymically and later (and still) as *Hemophilus influenzae* although it has no causal relation to that disease. Vaccine made from killed versions of the bacillus produced in the New York City Department of Health laboratories was used in Army camps and by large companies, including U.S. Steel, where some 289,000 employees were vaccinated.[65] The Army Medical School laboratories concentrated on vaccines against *Pneumococcus* and were using them in soldiers by October. *Streptococcus* was also regularly found in patients with influenza-related pneumonia, and the Puget Sound Navy Yard administered 33,000 doses of killed *Streptococci* to its sailors.

Contemporary recommendations were to empirically vaccinate against all those bacteria.[66] Edward Rosenow of the Mayo Clinic created a cocktail of killed versions of every one of them.[67] He gave it to 143,000 patients, and the Chicago Health Department used it on another 500,000. Rosenow circulated a questionnaire to the recipients asking how they had done and based on that questionable data he proclaimed his vaccine a success. Eventually a controlled study by George McCoy of the U.S. Public Health Service demonstrated that Rosenow's vaccine conferred no protection at all from influenza or its complications. Surgeon General Rupert Blue concluded that there was no evidence any of the vaccines worked, and he said all should be considered experimental only.[68]

An effective vaccine using inactive influenza virus was finally developed by Jonas Salk and Thomas Francis in the 1930s and was widely used by the U.S. military in World War II, but it was another decade before the Centers for Disease Control recommended its routine use in healthy young people. None of that helped the soldiers during the 1918 pandemic.

Soldiers in the camps proved an irresistible temptation for researchers. Experimental influenza vaccine was tested on 13,000 men at Camp Wheeler and another 12,000 at Camp Upton.[69] More aggressive experiments were carried out in Boston and San Francisco. At Boston's Deer Island training facility prisoners in the brig were offered pardon in return for participating in experiments in which mucous from influenza patients was painted in the back of their throats and blood from infected patients was injected under their skin. Experimental subjects held their faces close to those of patients and inhaled their breath for five minutes before having the patients cough in their faces. Each volunteer repeated this with ten different patients. Amazingly, of the sixty-two participants (thirty-nine of whom had no history of influenza), none became ill. Fifty sailors from the

Naval Training Station at Yerba Buena went through a similar set of experiments. None of them became ill either.[70]

Challenge trials in which volunteers are intentionally subjected to a communicable disease were obviously not new. Using soldiers as volunteers was not new either. It had been spectacularly effective in Cuba with yellow fever. A retrospective view of the influenza vaccine experiments was offered by Bradford Hale in a 1990 interview with the Therapeutic Trial Committee of the American Public Health Association. He testified that, "We did not ask the patient's permission or anybody's permission. We did not tell them we were in a trial—we just did it. To tell the truth, all of the discussion today about the *patient's* informed consent still strikes me as absolute rubbish."[71]

THE TOLL

The attitude about experimenting on humans changed dramatically after World War II, but the morbidity and mortality from influenza in 1918 pushed contemporary researchers to extraordinary lengths. In raw numbers the 1918 influenza was the greatest demographic disaster of the twentieth century and possibly of all human history. During the epidemic 47 percent of all deaths in the United States were from influenza, and average life expectancy in the country decreased by ten years.[72] Influenza killed more people in the United States than World War I, World War II, the Korean Conflict, and the Vietnam War combined.

Although there were fifteen civilian deaths for every death in the military, 26 percent of American soldiers caught influenza, and one in every sixty-seven died.[73] During the war there were 40,692,302 days lost to disease as opposed to 12,545,442 days lost to battle injury.[74] On any given day, the equivalent of six divisions was missing from the AEF due to disease, mostly influenza. In 1917 and 1918, 50,500 U.S. service members were killed in battle or died of combat wounds while 55,322 died of disease (mostly influenza) in Army camps, Navy installations, on transports, or in the AEF.[75]

In some ways American military medicine did very well in World War I. The admission rate in the U.S. Army for intestinal disease in 1861–62 was 29 times that in 1917–18, and the death rate was 258 times as high. In 1898–99 that incidence was 24 times as high, and the death rate was 125 times as high. Had the death rate from typhoid been the same in 1918 as in 1898, the Army would have lost 30,916 men to the disease. It lost 2,158.

Gorgas wanted the Great War to be the first in which loss of life in battle exceeded that from disease, and had it not been for influenza he would have gotten his wish. Both the admission and death rate for respiratory disease in 1917–18 were greater than that in either 1861–62 or 1898–99.[76] In a postwar report the surgeon general said: "Had it not been for influenza and pneumonia, the total rates (of infectious disease) for the years 1917–18 would have, indeed, been very small, both for admissions and for deaths."[77] For comparison, there only were nine deaths from influenza in the entire U.S. military between 1998 and 2014.[78]

It is impossible to arrive at the exact number of men who contracted influenza on the western front since many were treated in barracks or at the front and were not included in official reports. It is estimated, however, that the AEF had over 1 million cases, the British Expeditionary Force and the German Army had about 700,000 each, and the French Army about 436,000.[79] Both the incidence and mortality were significantly greater in the AEF than in the other armies. The reason for that is not certain, but the European armies had a high attack rate in the benign first wave and almost certainly carried immunity into the lethal second wave.

By the armistice the disease had largely run its course. There were scattered foci in January and February 1919, but neither the incidence nor the mortality approached that of late 1918. Cases broke out in American troops occupying Germany and in the expeditionary force at Archangel, which suffered 82 battle deaths but 2,352 hospitalizations and 104 deaths from influenza. There was also an outbreak in Paris during the peace conference. President Wilson got the disease in April, and there has been speculation that his lackluster performance at the Versailles peace negotiations may have been the result of his illness.

Demobilization and transport back to the United States may have spurred an outbreak in the spring of 1919, and in April when 9,428 men were in the hospital for injuries 44,172 men were still hospitalized for sickness.[80]

By late spring the pandemic ended. Perhaps the virus just ran out of susceptible hosts, although it is estimated that over 60 percent of the population would have had to have been infected for that to have occurred. H1N1 was replaced by other variants and did not reappear for half a century. What is clear is that medical care had nothing to do with it. The 1918 pandemic was a humbling and complete defeat for medical science just when the scientists thought they had finally gotten control of infectious disease.

CHAPTER 5

PHARMACOLOGY

Malaria and World War II

mallpox was the story of successful manipulation of immunity, and yellow fever was a triumphant exploitation of ecology to stop an epidemic. Typhoid deaths were the result of unnecessary failures of sanitation in successive wars, and influenza was a cautionary example of the failure of quarantine. In the early years of World War II there was a proven, effective drug to prevent and treat potentially lethal malaria. The problem was getting soldiers to use it.

MALARIA IN HISTORY

The viral pathogens we have looked at have been small and relatively simple, and recent advances in virology have brought our understanding of these organisms to the boundary between biology and chemistry. Malaria, on the other hand, is relatively large and vastly more complex.

Quarantine—separating hosts—has been used in malaria control but with decidedly mixed results. Sanitation—manipulating the environment by eliminating malaria's insect vector—has been difficult as *Anopheles* mosquitoes are both more widespread and more adaptable than their *Aedes* cousins. After years of research and a great deal of money spent there finally appears to be an effective vaccine, but that has only come in 2022. Fortunately, unlike the situation with viral epidemics, there has been a family of effective drugs, but they only work if they are taken, and that has been the military's problem.

During Marine stabilization operations in August 2003 in Liberia, 80 of the 290 troops who came ashore contracted malaria. Only 5 percent of the affected personnel had taken the antimalarial Mefloquine regularly, and only 14 percent of the entire force had blood levels of the drug high enough to afford protection against the disease.[1] To make matters worse only about a quarter of the Marines used DEET insect repellant because it was "too greasy," and none of the pyrethrum-treated mosquito nets they had been issued were even taken ashore. It is estimated that up to 100 percent of unprotected troops deployed in a future sub-Saharan action could be expected to contract malaria, and a U.S. military force in that area could well be rendered ineffective without a single combat engagement.[2]

We have seen repeatedly that when a war is complicated by an epidemic the battles enter cultural memory while diseases are largely forgotten. Malaria put more soldiers in the hospital than the Japanese in the Pacific War, but it remained largely invisible to the general public. In one bestselling account of the battle for Guadalcanal published in 1943, battles and skirmishes were described in vivid detail, but there was not a single mention of the malaria that nearly incapacitated the Marines and crippled the Japanese.[3]

The damage done by malaria leaves no fossil tracks, so the only sure evidence of the disease starts with the written word, and there have been descriptions of illnesses that sound like malaria as long as there has been writing. That is no surprise; the mosquitoes that spread the disease were here several million years before there were humans.

Sumerian documents from 6000–5500 BCE describe intermittent fevers in the flat, swampy Tigris and Euphrates basins. *Nei Ching*, the Chinese Canon of Medicine from 2700 BCE, describes fevers occurring every three or four days accompanied by enlargement of the spleen. The sixth-century BCE library of Ashurbanipal in Nineveh had accounts of malaria-like illness as did writing attributed to Hippocrates the following century. Alexander the Great may well have died of malaria in 323 BCE. The Romans were well acquainted with malaria, and both their armies and those of the Carthaginians were afflicted. Goths, Huns, and Lombards attacked Rome and were in turn attacked by malaria. Alaric probably died from malaria in 400 CE. Both Richard the Lion Heart and Saladin lost troops to fever in the swamps on the Palestinian coast and may have declared an armistice because of it. Chaucer and Shakespeare described what was likely malaria, and Dante died of it. Holy Roman Emperor Charles V succumbed to the disease in his monastery cell in Extremadura in 1558.

There was no malaria in the Americas before the English brought what was probably *vivax* to Jamestown. The Dutch and French brought *vivax* and the *malariae* variant to their colonies as well. *Falciparum* came with the slave trade that began in 1619.

The malaria incidence in early American wars is muddled by confused diagnoses and poor record-keeping, but incidence of malaria in the Civil War was probably considerable with more than 1.2 million episodes of what may have been malaria among Union and Confederate Armies with around eight thousand deaths.

Because America came late and fought almost entirely on the western front, malaria was not a significant problem for the U.S. Army in World War I, but such was not the case for the United Kingdom. In Macedonia the British Army had 168,751 admissions for malaria and evacuated 25,000 troops. Between October and December Field Marshal Edmund Allenby's troops in Syria had 20,000 cases and 773 deaths. The worst was in the East African Campaign where 57 percent of hospitalizations were for malaria with an annual admission rate of 1,423/1,000 troops.[4]

Of course, the impact of malaria is not only in times of conflict, and the disease remains ubiquitous. According to the World Health Organization, there were still 241 million cases of malaria with 627,000 deaths worldwide in 2020.[5]

THE DISEASE

The malaria organism is vastly more complicated than the viruses and salmonella we have looked at. Human malaria is caused by one of five *Plasmodia*: *falciparum, vivax, ovale, malariae,* and the more recently discovered and less frequent *knowlesi*. All invade red blood cells (RBCs) but have different preferences for cell type. *Falciparum* invades RBCs of all ages while *vivax* prefers reticulocytes and younger red cells. *Ovale* is virtually identical to *vivax,* and *malariae* prefers older cells. *Vivax* and *malariae* invade only 1–2 percent of RBCs and generally cause milder disease than *falciparum*, which can infect up to 40 percent of a host's total circulating red cell population.

Infected cells are more rigid than normal, and the spleen sees infected cells as degenerate and removes them from the bloodstream. Red cell sequestration and destruction cause profound anemia along with a swollen engorged spleen are hallmarks of malaria.

Intermittent fever starting eight to thirty days after a bite from an infected mosquito is the hallmark of malaria. *Falciparum* causes recurrent bouts of fever, typically forty-eight hours apart but sometimes chaotically spaced. Because of the forty-eight-hour interval and its lethality, *falciparum* was dubbed malignant tertian fever. *Vivax* is also on a three-day cycle, but being less lethal has been benign tertian fever, although as we shall see, "benign" is only relative. *Ovale* behaves very much like *vivax* while *malariae* recurs on a seventy-two-hour cycle. *Knowlesi*, which is usually seen in experimental settings, recurs with only a twenty-four-hour break between bouts. The exact cause of the fever is not certain, but it is probably related to coordinated release of interleukin-1 and tumor necrosis factor from circulating macrophages.

Clinically the disease resembles a viral infection with muscle aches and headaches and a fever of 103–105°F. Symptoms of gastroenteritis—nausea, vomiting, and diarrhea—are also common as is symptomatic hypoglycemia. *Falciparum* can cause much more serious diseases, especially in children who are more susceptible to cerebral infection, and 80 percent of current malaria deaths are from that cause. Massive lysis of RBCs can cause an outpouring of hemoglobin metabolites in the urine—black water fever—and renal failure. Release of cytokines can also result in pulmonary edema and hypoxia.

Prior infection with malaria results in only partial and generally short-lasting immunity, so recurrent infections are the rule rather than the exception. Fortunately recurrent infections are usually milder than the initial episode.

Malaria is anthropologically intriguing because the parasite appears to have driven human evolutionary change. Absence of the Duffy blood group antigen, a common condition in African Blacks, renders hosts relatively resistant to *Plasmodium vivax*. A single copy of the gene for sickle cell anemia (sickle cell trait) makes one unlikely to contract *falciparum* malaria, which is the dominant strain in much of Africa. Unfortunately two copies of the sickle gene result in full-blown sickle cell anemia, a debilitating and often fatal condition. Nature seems to have calculated that the risk of inheriting sickle cell disease in return for a population with only the trait and malaria resistance was a worthwhile trade. Thalassemia, relatively common in the Mediterranean, also confers protection as does a genetic deficiency in glucose-6-phosphate dehydrogenase.

A susceptible human host is only half of what is necessary for propagation of malaria; the parasite requires a mosquito vector, and the plasmodial life story is a fascinating one. The cycle begins and ends in the same place so we will start with a mosquito bite. But first a bit about the biter.

THE MOSQUITOES

There are roughly 460 species of *Anopheles* mosquitoes, and more than 100 of them can transmit human malaria. Females lay up to two hundred eggs on water although species vary as to what kind of water they prefer—fresh or brackish, still or running, in shade or in full sun. Over the next ten to fourteen days, the eggs morph into larvae and then pupae before emerging as adults. Only the females feed on blood, which they require to produce eggs. A female *Anopheles* only lives for a couple of weeks, but unlike the *Aedes* who stay close to home, she can travel up to a mile and a half during her short life.

Other mosquitoes land softly with their body parallel to the host and almost gently lower their proboscis into the skin, but *Anopheles* aggressively puts its head down, hoists its body nearly vertical, and hits like a dart. While feeding she injects small bits of saliva to keep the blood flowing, and in the process injects tiny malarial sporozoites into the bloodstream.

The blood-borne sporozoites congregate in the liver where one of two things happens. Some of them mature into liver schizonts each of which can release 10,000 to 30,000 merozoites back into the bloodstream to hunt for new host RBCs. If the invader is *vivax* some of the sporozoites stay behind in the liver and go dormant. These hypnozoites lurk for months and even years before waking up and going into the bloodstream to cause a new

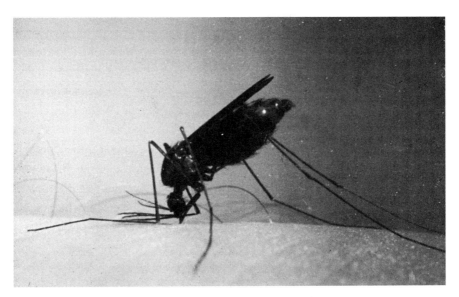

Anopheles **mosquito, the malaria vector** *National Library of Medicine*

bout of clinical malaria. That does not happen with *falciparum*, which only causes disease once in each infection.

The merozoites in the bloodstream seek out and invade RBCs where they mature into ring and trophozoite forms that can be seen with the proper stain and a good microscope. Eventually infected RBCs packed with merozoites rupture, and infectious particles pour into the bloodstream in search of new RBCs to infect. That process occurs with remarkable synchronicity and coincides with the clinical bouts of fever. Some merozoites also mature into male and female gametocytes, which are the only ones able to continue the malarial cycle outside the human host.

Now the *Anopheles* reenters the picture. She bites an infected host and ingests the male and females gametocytes that then come together as zygotes that make oocysts capable of producing more than ten thousand new sporozoites that find their way to the mosquito salivary gland, and the cycle is ready to repeat. In all it takes from nine to seventeen days from the first bite until the mosquito is ready to transmit the disease again. If you have been keeping count, you might remember that the average female mosquito's lifespan is only a couple of weeks, so many of them die before being able to transmit the disease, but some do not.

The discovery that mosquitoes were a necessary link in the transmission of malaria and the complex steps in that process was not a triumph of American medicine, but it was very much the work of British and French military surgeons. The first clue came from Italian physician Giovanni Rasori who suggested that it was a parasite and not bad air (*mal 'aria*) that was responsible for transmission of the disease. The real story began in 1866 when newly minted Scottish physician Patrick Manson took a position as medical officer to the Chinese Imperial Customs on Formosa and had his first exposure to the tropical diseases that became his life's work. Manson spent five years in Formosa and another thirteen in the coastal city of Amoy (now Xiamen) where a variety of tropical infectious diseases, especially malaria, were hyperendemic.

Manson was a meticulous observer. Dissection and microscopic examination of mosquitoes fed on a Chinese patient's limb swollen and distorted by elephantiasis (filariasis) revealed the causative organism and gave Manson his first proven disease with an insect vector. His elephantiasis paper read before the Linnean Society of London in 1878 was met with less than universal acclaim. One critic said, "what they had heard represented either the work of a genius or more likely the emanations of a drunken Scottish doctor in far-off China where, everyone was aware, they drank far too much whiskey."[6]

In 1894 Manson was back in London. He was convinced that mosquitoes were also responsible for transmission of malaria, but there was no malaria in London, and Manson needed someone working where the disease was endemic to carry on his work.

Meanwhile Charles Louis Laveran was looking at humans, the other step in the transmission of the disease. Military medicine was the Laveran family business. His father was an army surgeon and had been a professor in the military hospital at Val-de-Grace. His mother's father and grandfather were both senior officers in the French Army. Laveran was born in Paris, raised in Algeria, and trained in medicine and public health at Strasbourg. He followed in his father's footsteps as Chairman of Military Diseases and Epidemics at Val-de-Grace before being posted back to Algeria from 1878 to 1883 where he first saw the malarial parasite in the blood of a febrile soldier.

Although he later denied it, Laveran likely was aware of Manson's mosquito theory. Besides, there are doubts about whether it was even possible to see the parasite with the microscope Laveran used. At any rate he went on to the Italian campagna where there was an abundance of malaria cases, he got a better microscope, and the parasites he was looking for proved ubiquitous.

Laveran spent the next twenty-seven years studying protozoal diseases and working either on active duty or as a consultant to the French military including a stint advising the Army on malaria control during World War I. He was awarded the Nobel Prize in Physiology or Medicine in 1907 primarily for his work on trypanosomiasis, another protozoal disease. Laveran gave half the money from that prize to establish the Laboratory in Tropical Medicine at the Pasteur Institute.

While Laveran was working on malaria in humans, Manson found the collaborator he needed to continue his mosquito work. Ronald Ross was the oldest of ten children of General Sir C. C. G. Ross. His father wanted him to join the army, but the younger Ross was intent on being either a poet, an artist, or both. Ross spent his life drawing and painting and published several plays and volumes of poetry that were well-received at the time but have held up poorly. They also failed to earn him a living.

As a compromise the general sent his son to St. Bartholomew's Hospital to study medicine, intending for him to be a military surgeon. Ross was a mediocre student at best, and it took him two tries to pass the licentiate examination for the Society of Apothecaries, the least prestigious of Britain's three available medical credentials. Bowing to his father's wishes, he spent four months at the Army Medical School before joining the Indian Medical Service.

In the beginning Ross was as lackluster a physician as he had been a student, remaining more interested in poetry than disease, but on sabbatical in London in 1888 and 1889 he got a diploma in public health from the Royal College of Physicians and the Royal College of Surgeons and took a course in bacteriology. That piqued his interest.

Ross was convinced that malaria came from an intestinal bacteria until he met Manson on a second trip to London in 1894. Manson convinced

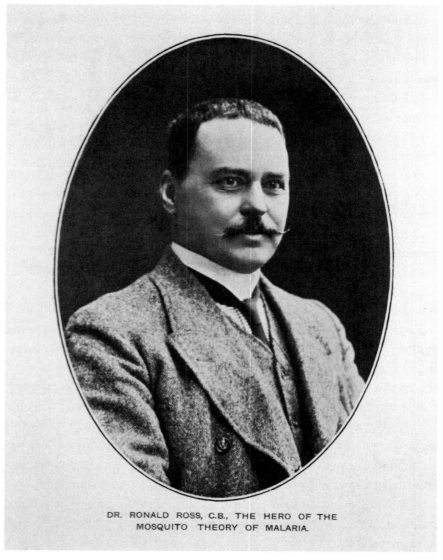

DR. RONALD ROSS, C.B., THE HERO OF THE
MOSQUITO THEORY OF MALARIA.

Sir Ronald Ross, the British military surgeon who worked out the life cycle of the malaria parasite *National Library of Medicine*

him of the mosquito hypothesis, and Ross set out to prove it when he returned to India in 1895. For the next two and half years he dissected one insect after another, but the only thing he got out of that was his own case of malaria. He had been looking at the wrong mosquitoes.

Finally, more by luck than intent, Ross stumbled on *Anopheles* and found plasmodia in the mosquito's abdomen. That led to reports in the *Indian Medical Journal* in 1897 and in the *British Medical Journal* the same year. He picked mosquitoes apart with needles futilely hunting for parasites that could be transmitted by a bite until he finally looked in the salivary glands and found them packed with parasites. Ross had the progression from the mosquito gut to the salivary glands. The next obvious steps were from the salivary gland to the proboscis to the human, but he never finished the proof. In addition Ross' work was done on avian malaria, and he did not bother to prove that the cycle was the same in the human disease.

That was left to Giovanni Grassi and his coworkers Amico Bignami and Giovanni Bastianelli who discovered *Plasmodium vivax* and described the clinical stages of that form as well as *falciparum* and *malariae*. By 1898 Grassi had proven that female *Anopheles* mosquitoes were the vectors of human disease. As with yellow fever, there was more than a little possessiveness among the Italians for *their* disease. After all Italy had Europe's highest malaria incidence and had for millennia, and Italian scientists thought it presumptuous of the French and English to think they had solved what was clearly an Italian problem.

The fight over precedence peaked in 1902 when the Nobel Prize for Physiology or Medicine was awarded. The committee initially intended the prize to go jointly to Ross and Grassi, but Ross went on the offensive. He accused Grassi of fraud, and the committee appointed Robert Koch to be an "impartial" arbiter. The German professor was not fond of Italians and came down firmly in favor of Ross who was awarded the prize alone.

Ross' rancor was not limited to Grassi. He was jealous of Manson's fame and attacked him as well. Although he had written Manson 110 times while in India and received 85 replies and even wrote that the mosquito discoveries were to his credit alone, Ross did not once mention Manson in his Nobel acceptance speech.

Ross continued to publish purplish prose as well as erudite mathematical studies of the epidemiology of infectious diseases. He lost a son in World War I and served with the Royal Army Medical Corps in Alexandria, where he studied dysentery in the troops returning from Gallipoli. He died respected but generally unloved in 1932.

THE DRUGS

By the turn of the century, the malarial life cycle was worked out, and even better there was an effective treatment. For an uncertain but considerable time before Europeans came to South America Incas had used bark from the cinchona tree to treat muscle spasms and shivering from cold exposure. In 1636 a Jesuit priest trained as an apothecary guessed that bark that controlled shaking might be of use in malaria, and he sent samples home to be tested. "Jesuit bark" became standard treatment for malaria and a variety of other fevers and became one of the New World's most valuable exports. In 1820 Joseph Pelletier and Joseph Bienaimé Caventou isolated quinine and proved it was the active ingredient in cinchona bark.

The Spanish in Peru made a futile effort to maintain a monopoly on cinchona. First the British tried to sneak seeds out and grow them in India in 1859, but the trees failed to produce useful bark. The Dutch, however, also purloined cinchona seeds and sent them to the East Indies and eventually set up the Kina Bureau, an Amsterdam cartel to import, process, store, and sell quinine. By the 1930s their plantations in Java were generating 22 million pounds of cinchona bark a year and 97 percent of the world's quinine.

Ironically, the Dutch quinine monopoly played a major role in Germany's emergence as an industrial power. That story began in the middle of the nineteenth century with William Perkin, a nineteen-year-old student at the Royal College of Chemistry in London. British industrial entrepreneurs had recently found that igniting the vapors from burning coal gave off useful light, a discovery that was the death knell of the whale oil industry. The residuum left when coal gas vaporized was a fascinating chemical soup. While trying to make quinine out of the mess Perkin got a brilliant red powder. He then experimented with the aniline sludge left after naphtha had been extracted, created a mauve dye, and became rich. That artificial color was followed shortly by other reds, blues, greens, and violets.

British academicians met the discovery with general indifference. Not so the Germans. Chemists at BASF, Hoechst, Bayer, and Agfa dove into chemical dyes and from there into drugs derived from them, and Germany became a powerhouse of industrial chemistry.

Before we follow that story further, a word about quinine itself. The drug impairs the ability of merozoites inside RBCs to metabolize hemoglobin,

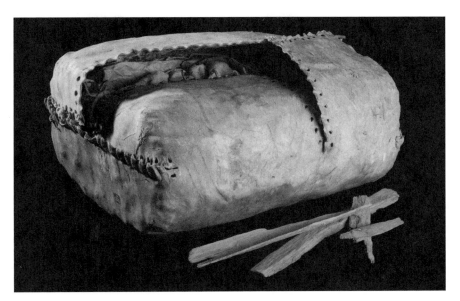

Bag of cinchona bark, the source of quinine, which was still a primary treatment for malaria in World War II *Wellcome Library*

but it has no effect on the gametocytes that go back into mosquitoes and allow the disease to be transmitted. Still, in high doses quinine can stop an acute malaria attack and cure some cases of *falciparum* malaria, especially if given intravenously. It also suppresses *vivax* and *malariae* disease, but only as long as it is taken. When the drug is stopped the schizonts sheltering in the liver reemerge as does the disease. Quinine also has a short half-life; its plasma concentration drops 90 percent in just twenty-four hours.

And the drug has several unpleasant side effects. At therapeutic doses tinnitus, hearing loss, vertigo, headaches, nausea, and visual difficulty are common. Other side effects are less common but can be lethal. Angioneurotic edema, heart rhythm irregularities (long QT syndrome), diffuse intravascular coagulation, thrombotic thrombocytopenia purpura, and renal failure are all potentially deadly. Nonetheless, as the only treatment for malaria and one of the only effective treatments for any infectious disease for centuries, quinine was invaluable.

There was, however, a supply problem in World War II. After the May 1940 invasion of the Netherlands control of the Kina Bureau was transferred to Bandung in the East Indies, but quinine production virtually ceased after the Japanese took the Dutch colonies in March 1942. The United States had stockpiled cinchona and quinine before the war, but supplies were not nearly enough to support military action in the Pacific, Southeast Asia, Africa, and Southern Europe, all of which had endemic malaria.

Collection of quinine supplies was one of the great medical oddities of the war. It was common practice in mid-century America for pharmacies to compound their own proprietary medicines, and quinine was regularly included in cold medicines and other concoctions. In December 1942, the National Research Council called for voluntary pooling of all retail stocks of quinine under supervision of the American Pharmaceutical Association into a National Quinine Pool. Pharmacies across the country were asked to send in all powder, tablets, and capsules of quinine, quinidine cinchonine, cinchonidine, and salts of any of them. The pool was happy to accept either full or open bottles, and what came in was sorted and crushed into powder that yielded 13 million five-gram doses of quinine. The program continued until October 1943 by which time quinine was effectively replaced by Atabrine.[7]

When the Germans campaigning in hyperendemic East Africa in World War I lost access to quinine, their chemists started a frantic search for synthetic quinine. After a series of failures Bayer came up with pamaquine naphthoate (Plasmochin) in 1925. The drug was effective against malaria but caused abdominal and back pain and turned patients blue-gray (probably from methemoglobinemia) and was considered too toxic to be used outside the hospital.[8] Plasmochin was followed in 1930 by less dangerous quinacrine (Mepacrine, Atabrine).

German chemists also created Sontochin, the formula for which was smuggled to the United States by Vichy French physicians after the fall of Tunis in 1943. With minor modifications that drug became chloroquine, which was identical to another German drug that had been abandoned as too toxic for human use. After adjusting the dose and schedule of administration chloroquine became the standard malaria treatment for several decades, but all that was too late to be of use in World War II.

Chloroquine also proved useful in amebiasis, lupus erythematosus, and rheumatoid arthritis and resurfaced in 2021 as an unproven therapy for COVID-19. Santoquine (French), Proguanil (British), and Primaquine

(United States) came from studies of more than 15,000 compounds evaluated in the 1940s, but all came too late to be used during the war.[9]

Atabrine was the mainstay. World War II would be the first time an "Atabrinized" army would fight in malaria-ridden areas, but acceptance of malaria prophylaxis was anything but automatic. Circular Letter No. 56 issued by the Office of the Surgeon General on June 9, 1941, stated, "The use of quinine or Atabrine for prophylaxis is not recommended as a routine procedure as the available information indicates that these drugs do not prevent infection. However, they are of definite military value in that they do prevent the appearance of the clinical symptoms of malaria as long as they are taken."[10] The half-hearted endorsement may have been related to the fact that quinine stocks were predicted to be used up in less than two years. Quinine would be used sparingly and mostly to treat acute disease until Atabrine solved the shortage problem in the spring of 1944.

Atabrine's primary action is against the asexual erythrocytic parasites, and like quinine it is ineffective against gametocytes. Nonetheless, a loading dose can abort acute attacks. The drug lingers in white cells, the liver, spleen, lungs, and heart, and unlike quinine 50 percent of the original dose is still present a week after the last dose. If suppression is continued long enough and if the parasite is not resistant, *falciparum* disease can be cured with Atabrine. The same is not true of *vivax*, which typically recurs four to six weeks after the last dose.

Atabrine has a few real side effects and several that were fallaciously attributed to it. Rumor and Japanese propaganda led to widespread belief that the drug caused impotence, sterility, or both. It did neither. In high doses the drug did cause transient mild gastrointestinal upset, but because it was often started just before men boarded ships for amphibious operations Atabrine was also blamed for a combination of anxiety and seasickness. The rumors were pervasive enough that articles about Atabrine were kept out of Australian newspapers likely to be read by Allied soldiers.

One side effect was real. Atabrine was from a family of quinolone dyes, and it did turn men a sickly yellow. Rumors that the yellow color was from liver damage were, however, false.

Atabrine did have other rare but significant side effects. It is a cerebral cortical stimulant, and there were occasional associated psychoses.

Atypical lichen planus—a flat white rash of the skin and mucous membranes—and aplastic anemia were uncommon complications.

Much of the Atabrine problem was lack of information about the correct dose and administration schedule. The drug would eventually be the model for dose-response studies, but that would take a while. When the war started little was known about the absorption, excretion, or blood levels of Atabrine, and it was uncertain whether there would be bad effects from taking the drug for prolonged periods. There was also concern that Atabrine produced in the United States had contaminants not present in the drug made by German pharmaceutical companies. The American military had tried the drug in Panama in 1938, but there was no organized study of how much to give and when to give it. In the Canal Zone Atabrine proved less effective at both preventing and treating malaria than quinine and was abandoned.

If the initial dose was too low the drug accumulated in the muscle and liver and never achieved a blood level high enough to be effective. Early on "QAP therapy" was the standard mash-up. Totaquine (a mixture of quinine-like drugs) was given until the fever was controlled. Then there were five days of high-dose Atabrine followed by two days of rest then five days of Plasmochin. It was eventually found that one gram of Atabrine a week was enough to prevent 98 percent of clinical disease but giving most of that on the first day caused gastrointestinal side effects and an unacceptable number of psychotic episodes. It had to be spread out.

In the first years of the war every military surgeon was free to try his own Atabrine schedule, and no one collected data on how the various regimens compared in either safety or effectiveness. Military physicians—especially those in the Marines—did not trust the drug and refused to prescribe it. They substituted quinine or nothing. Systematic studies were finally started in late 1942, and, by mid-1943, one hundred milligrams every day was standard.

Atabrine was a German invention, and German companies with a U.S. patent had licensed production and sale to the Winthrop Chemical Company. Under Executive Order No. 9193 issued July 6, 1942, the Alien Property Custodian was given authority "to control, manage, or vest" all foreign interest in patents, and all matters relevant to production of Atabrine were given to the custodian. Royalty-free license to produce the drug was distributed among eleven companies for the duration of the war plus six months. Winthrop alone produced 2.5 billion doses of Atabrine by the end of the war.[11]

THE WAR

Malaria was a problem in most theaters of World War II. The disease was a major factor in the Philippines, in the South and Southwest Pacific, in China and Southeast Asia, in Africa, and in southern Europe. The experience in the various areas was different enough that we need to deal with them separately.

The Philippines

Malaria first struck U.S. forces in the Philippines. The archipelago comprises over seven thousand islands, although only eleven account for 94 percent of the land mass. The islands' average temperature is 80°F and varies little from season to season. The warm, wet climate is ideal for *Anopheles*, and the Philippines have thirty-two resident species four of which carry malaria. There were an estimated 1–2 million active cases of malaria in the islands when the Japanese invaded.

That invasion started ten hours after the Pearl Harbor attack with the destruction of the American air forces at Clark Field. On December 22, the Japanese 14th Army under Lieutenant General Masahuru Homma sailed south from nearby Formosa and landed on Luzon with orders to conquer the island within fifty days. Gen. Douglas MacArthur intended to resist the Japanese wherever they landed but, when Filipino forces were easily pushed back at Lingayen Gulf and no sea or air support was forthcoming, he withdrew to the Bataan Peninsula across the bay from Manila and to the fortified island of Corregidor. Bataan is 450 square miles jutting south between Manila Bay and the South China Sea and is one of the most infected areas of the malarious Philippines.

MacArthur's decision was made in haste, and the retreat was chaotic. Enough rice to feed 105,000 people for five months, 3,400,000 gallons of fuel, 500,000 rounds of ammunition, and almost all medical supplies were left in Cabanatuan.[12] The armies took only enough rice for twenty days and almost no medicine. After the withdrawal Bataan held 83,000 American and Filipino troops and 26,000 civilians who resisted 75,000 Japanese for the next three months. Many in the retreat were without shoes, blankets, underwear, and—perhaps most importantly—mosquito nets.[13]

MacArthur only visited Bataan once after the invasion. On January 9, he told the troops that they should be able to hold out for several months and that help was on the way. Then he went back to Corregidor. He left for Australia March 12 after having received $500,000 from Philippine President Manuel Quezon as "recompense and reward" for his services and was given the Medal of Honor for his defense of Bataan on March 26.

The conditions he left on the peninsula were horrific. Rations were initially cut to two thousand calories a day, then one thousand, then close to zero. By March 80 percent of the defenders on Bataan were unfit for duty, and seven thousand were hospitalized.[14] Every day five hundred new cases of malaria were admitted to hospitals.[15] One million quinine tablets were found on Cebu and shipped to Bataan, but they were not enough to treat active cases much less provide prophylaxis. Lethal cerebral malaria spread after quinine supplies were exhausted.

The Japanese suffered as well. The 14th Army had 10,000 to 12,000 cases of malaria—at one point was down to 3,000 effective fighters—and reinforcements had to be transferred from Singapore. The numbers of battle injuries were small in comparison. In the end the Japanese took the Philippines having lost only three thousand killed and five thousand wounded.

Despite their hopeless situation and the lack of support from the United States, on February 9 President Franklin Roosevelt ordered the Army not to surrender. Out of food, out of medicine, and out of soldiers healthy enough to fight, Maj. Gen. Edward King disobeyed and surrendered on April 8. It was—if one does not count Quebec in the Revolution—the first time an American army had surrendered in a foreign war. Former Secretary of War General Patrick Hurley said, "We were out-shipped, out-planed, out-manned and out-gunned by the Japanese."[16] An army surgeon put it differently: "The capitulation of Luzon force represents in many respects a defeat due to disease and starvation rather than military conditions. Malnutrition, malaria, and intestinal infections had reduced the combat efficiency of our forces more than 75 percent."[17] Both were correct.

It was a humiliation, but the defenders had stretched the inevitable defeat out for three months—two months more than the British held out in Malaya. A month after Bataan surrendered, Corregidor did the same. But that was also the month of the Battle of the Coral Sea when the tide of war in the Pacific began to turn.

For the men of Bataan the ordeal was just beginning. They faced the brutal march to prisoner-of-war camps where they spent the next three and a half years, and malaria accompanied them every step of the way. When they surrendered they had at least 24,000 active cases of malaria. It was mostly *vivax*, which without suppression would recur over and over again.[18] Of the almost 29,589 deaths at Camp O'Donnell in 1942, 6,179 were from malaria. At Cabanatuan 25 percent of the deaths were from malaria. The Japanese supplied quinine but not enough to treat the acute cases, and there was nothing for prophylaxis.[19]

Bataan was a brutal lesson in malaria. All the disease needed to become epidemic was a susceptible host population—preferably crowded and depleted—the right kind of mosquitoes, and no effective prevention or treatment. Bataan met all those requirements, and malaria had a field day. Although the same conditions would be met in other theaters it took two years and tens of thousands of lost lives for the lesson to sink in.

China-Burma-India

Malaria next struck in the China-Burma-India Theater, an area spanning 2,400 miles east to west and 1,800 miles north to south and encompassing over 2 million square miles. Burma (now Myanmar) alone covered 416,000 square miles, largely jungle and almost entirely malarious. Mountains rising ten thousand feet separate the flat Irrawaddy plain from India to the west and China to the east. The British colonized Burma in 1824 and ruled it as part of India until 1937 when it was made a separate colony. After the Japanese seized eastern China the only land route to supply Kunming where Chiang Kai-shek and his Nationalist forces headquarters was a seven-hundred-mile dirt road over the mountains from Burma.

Malaria was rampant in the entire area. In 1941, India had 100 to 200 million cases out of a total population of 388 million, and the disease was responsible for up to one and a half million deaths a year. It was by far the most important disease in that country. Burmese towns were far worse with a death rate of 214/1,000 in 1939 alone.[20] It was virtually impossible to separate military forces operating in the area from residents infected with malaria, especially since many of the locals provided manual labor for the armies. Mosquito control and suppression of malaria were nonexistent in India before 1944. The biggest spikes in incidence were in July 1943 and 1944 when troops operating in the theater had an incidence of over 300/1,000 a year.[21]

After quick victories in the Netherlands East Indies, Singapore, and Malaya the Japanese surprised the British by sending two divisions north into Burma from Siam (Thailand) on January 20, 1942. Japanese troops routed two inexperienced British divisions and their Indian and Burmese allies. When they took Rangoon on March 8, the land communication to Kunming was severed.

Maj. Gen. William Slim took command of forces in the theater with American Lt. Gen. Joseph Stilwell in charge of American and American-trained Chinese forces. Slim crossed into India from Burma in May 1942 in a retreat that cost the Allies 13,000 casualties along with 50,000 civilian deaths and creation of 500,000 Burmese refugees at a cost of only 4,000 casualties for the Japanese. Stilwell told reporters, "We got run out of Burma and it is humiliating as hell."[22]

American military leaders still believed China was key to defeating Japan, and their options for keeping the Nationalist Army fighting were limited. They could supply Kunming by flying air transports over the 15,000-foot Himalayas, an altitude that stressed both the planes and the pilots. They could try to retake the Burmese end of the road to China and reopen it, or they could try to retake Burma altogether. The China-Burma-India Theater was officially organized March 4, 1942, to attempt one or more of those strategies.

The British were unenthusiastic about opening the road, and in late 1942 they launched a limited ground invasion of a strip of western Burma including Akyab Island. The island had airstrips the British command thought might be used to attack and eventually retake Rangoon and pro-tect Calcutta. The force was undersupplied, riddled with malaria, and soundly defeated.

Chiang Kai-shek wanted money, aircraft, and armaments to ensure his position relative to rival Chinese warlords. He demanded three American divisions, five hundred airplanes, and five thousand tons of supplies a month all of which would have to be flown in "over the Hump," but he had no intention of sending Chinese troops to Burma.

Americans serving in the theater were convinced that neither the British nor the Indians were especially interested in fighting the Japanese. They were correct; at the January 1943 Casablanca conference the British announced that troops and supplies would not be available to retake Burma before the end of 1944. After the Arcadia Conference American and British resources were committed to defeating Germany. American GIs joked that C-B-I stood for "Confused Bastards in India" and SEAC (Southeast Asia Command) was short for "Save England's Asian Colonies." General Sir Archibald Wavell and Stilwell briefly considered launching a Burma campaign in late 1942, but the diversion of virtually all resources to the belabored British in North Africa scotched that idea.

As an alternative to a real invasion Wavell formed the 77th Long-Range Penetration Brigade under eccentric Brigadier Orde Wingate who had previously served with commando units in Palestine and Ethiopia. Small groups of men dispersed deep into Burma could be resupplied by air and operating independently could sabotage key Japanese assets in the country.

Japanese soldiers thought Burma was the worst posting in the whole Empire, and Wingate set out to prove them right. His three-thousand-man brigade was nicknamed Chindits after the half lion, half eagle *Chenthe* that adorned Buddhist temples. They operated over 1,500 miles of Burmese jungle for three months and proved for the first time that Western soldiers could function in the jungle just as well as the Japanese. Their strategic and even tactical significance was limited, but the Chindits were a propaganda triumph.

That triumph was very nearly prevented by a catastrophic outbreak of malaria. Slim said, "In 1943 for every man evacuated with wounds, we had one hundred twenty evacuated sick. . . . A simple calculation showed me that in a matter of months at this rate my army would have melted away. Indeed, it was doing so under my eyes."[23] It was no exaggeration. The attack rate among forward troops in Burma was 12/1,000 *per day*. At that rate Slim's entire army would have been gone in three months.[24]

Wingate's Chindits took great pride in not caring for themselves. They were tough commandos trained to operate deep behind enemy lines; disease prevention was beneath them. Their officers thought hard training and physical endurance were all that was needed to prevent malaria. The Chindits cut off their pant legs, rolled up their sleeves, and refused mosquito repellant. They were issued jungle hammocks with mosquito netting that could be zipped at night, but they refused to carry them. The nets weighed seven pounds, shut off air circulation in the steaming jungle nights, and would be hard to get out of in the event of a surprise Japanese attack.

Almost no one bothered with Mepacrine (Atabrine). Within six weeks 70 percent of the Chindits were hospitalized with malaria, and the average soldier had up to seven attacks. In February 1943 three thousand Chindits were sent to Burma for four months in Operation Longcloth. Only six hundred of them were ever fit to serve again.

Mepacrine avoidance was not peculiar to the Chindits. Military physicians in India were skeptical of the drug as well. The ones who thought it worked worried that it would conceal infection and encourage officers to keep sick men on duty. In the case of *vivax* malaria they were right; the drug was meant to keep men fighting, not to cure them. Officers thought (without evidence) the drug would decrease fighting efficiency, and the ranks believed rumors of Mepacrine caused impotence. Routine Mepacrine suppression was not used in Burma until early 1944, and then only when a unit's commander deemed it necessary.[25]

Slim knew better and had a solution. He staged surprise inspections of his units to see if the men were taking the drug. "If the overall result was less than ninety-five percent positive, I sacked the commanding officer. I only had to sack three; by then the rest had got my meaning."[26] Lieutenant General Sir Neil Cantlie said this was the first time in history that any combatant officer who allowed his men to become ineffective because of disease was deemed unfit for command.[27] By 1945 the malaria incidence among British soldiers was down to 1/1,000 per day, a sick rate Slim pointed out was lower than that of the average worker in London.[28]

Wingate showed up at the August 1943 Quebec Conference and mes-merized senior American military leaders. They agreed to fund a new Chindit expedition into Burma and authorized creation of an American commando force to join them. The 5307th Provisional Regiment, code-named Galahad and commanded by Brig. Gen. Frank Merrill who had been with Stilwell during the 1942 Burma rout, was the first American ground combat unit in the C-B-I theater. Thanks to a *Time Life* reporter they became Merrill's Marauders. The men were recruited from veterans of jungle warfare in the South Pacific along with a variety of psychologically questionable misfits and more than a few who volunteered believing a short tour in Burma would get them sent home. When the Marauders came to Bombay in October 1943 the plan was for them to serve with the Chindits, but Stilwell would have none of it. He insisted they operate independently. The Office of Strategic Services did train Kachin tribesmen, historic ene-mies of the Bamar Burmese, as scouts and guides for the Marauders.

Stilwell planned to send the men from Ledo to India to reopen the Burma Road. The plan was to take the airstrip outside Myitkyina and then the town itself. Painful experience taught the British that malaria could be managed, but the Americans had yet to learn that lesson. Stilwell's malaria expert found one unit with an attack rate of 4,080/1,000 per year. Even though the unit had become useless in combat there remained little inter-est in malaria prevention.

The men hated mosquito netting for the same reasons the Chindits had. They found mosquito repellant too greasy; besides it stained clothes and dissolved plastic. The repellant may have been the only war resource for which the supply was greater than the demand.

In February 1944, 2,750 men of the 5307th went into Burma. Every man was expected to take Atabrine daily on the schedule worked out in the Southwest Pacific, but as soon as they were in Burma the men stopped tak-ing the drug. The unit fought two more or less successful battles with the Japanese 18th Division before taking the airstrip at Myitkyina. Then things turned sour. Merrill, already suffering from malaria, had a heart attack and had to be evacuated.[29] The men were exhausted, and seventy-five to one hundred of them were being evacuated for illness every day. Men with fevers were discharged from the hospital and sent straight back to combat.

Detailed descriptions of the campaign only mention malaria in passing even though the disease was the reason it took the combined American and Chinese forces more than three months to take the town of Myitkyina.[30] By the time the town fell only two hundred of the original unit were still active. What remained of the 3507th was dissolved, and the remnant was absorbed into the 475th Infantry, the predecessor of the modern 75th Ranger Regiment.

The Japanese suffered as well although medical records are lacking. Prisoners of war told their captors that every Japanese soldier had malaria at least once, that 30 percent were sick at any one time, and that some of them had as many as fifteen attacks.[31]

Ironically, by the time Myitkyina fell Burma was a sideshow in a theater that had become largely irrelevant. The Japanese Fifteenth Army under Lieutenant General Renya Mutaguchi had attempted an invasion of India and suffered a catastrophic defeat at Imphal in March 1944. The invaders sustained 60,000 casualties in the empire's worst land defeat of the war. For once combat caused more casualties than disease in Southeast Asia.

The British were deeply concerned that a Japanese invasion would rob them of their Indian empire. The Americans thought the Nationalist Army would be a formidable ally and that retaking eastern China was vital to defeating Japan. Neither turned out to be true. In the end the China-Burma-India theater was as much a story of disease as of warfare and had little effect on the war's outcome.

At least by the time the theater became irrelevant Allied military leaders had come to understand how serious malaria was. Atabrine was mandatory in Assam, East Bengal, and Burma by early 1945, and the spring and summer rates in the "Atabrine zone" stabilized at 15 to 20/1,000 per year, a fraction of what they had been two years earlier.[32]

The Southwest Pacific

Roosevelt called China-Burma-India in the east and Australia in the west the two "vital flanks" in the war with Japan. The eastern flank turned out not to be so vital, but the struggle to maintain open access to Australia was almost the entire American focus for the first two years of the Pacific War. Great Britain assumed primary responsibility for the area from Singapore to Suez. Australia and New Zealand each had modest military forces, and they had to protect their home countries. The Dutch and French were out of the war. That left the United States to roll back Japanese advances, but first they had to secure sea routes between America and Australia.

In March 1942, MacArthur was in Melbourne and had assumed command of slowly growing allied forces in the southwest Pacific. Although the European theater would eventually assume priority, 80,000 U.S. troops were moved to the Southwest Pacific between January and March with 210,000 more scheduled before the end of the year.[33]

MacArthur had a formidable reputation and assumed he would be in command of the Pacific theater, but the admirals thought differently. Most of them had a low opinion of the general and were profoundly unenthusiastic about having him command their fleet, so an ungainly compromise divided the theater into two parts. MacArthur would be in charge of Australia, the Philippines, the Solomon Islands, New Guinea, the Bismarck Archipelago, Borneo, and all of the Dutch East Indies except Sumatra. The Navy under Adm. Ernest King got the rest of the Pacific save coastal waters off Central and South America. Vice Adm. Robert L. Ghormley was King's commander of the South Pacific Area.

MacArthur had little time to object. On March 8, the Japanese landed at Huon Gulf in eastern New Guinea. The immediate worry was that the Japanese meant to use New Guinea as a staging area to invade Australia. The Imperial High Command had briefly considered that but rejected the invasion as beyond their manpower and supply resources. Instead they intended to take Port Moresby on the south coast of New Guinea and use it as a base to harass northern Australia and the sea lanes to North America. To that end the Japanese also intended to take New Caledonia, the Fiji Islands, and Samoa. Taking eastern New Guinea, Papua, and the Solomons would also protect their large bases at Rabaul and Truk Island.

A major amphibious attack was stopped at the Battle of the Coral Sea May 4–8, technically fought within MacArthur's area of control but conducted by Adm. Chester Nimitz's carrier task force. The Japanese lost only the small carrier *Shoho* and suffered damage to the larger carrier *Shokaku*. U.S. losses were more severe. The carrier USS *Lexington* was sunk along with the destroyer USS *Sims* and the oiler *Neosho*. Even though the

U.S. Navy suffered heavier losses, the Japanese abandoned the landing, and Port Moresby was temporarily spared.

New Guinea is 1,500 miles long and 400 miles across at its widest and is shaped like a peacock with the head pointing north and west and a long tail draping south and east. Mountains run in a spine from one end to the other, and, although the western end of the island is on the equator, the mountains are high enough to have year-round snow caps. South of the spine a jungle swamp merges into steep rainforest. Both the terrain and the climate are forbidding, and less than 1 percent of the island was under cultivation in 1942. The average temperature in the lowlands is 80°F. Port Moresby, on the south coast of the bird's tail, is relatively dry with only forty inches of rain a year, but in the foothills the average is seven times that.

The jungles at the mountain bases are ideal for malaria-carrying *Anopheles favanti*, and both *falciparum* and *vivax* malaria are prevalent,

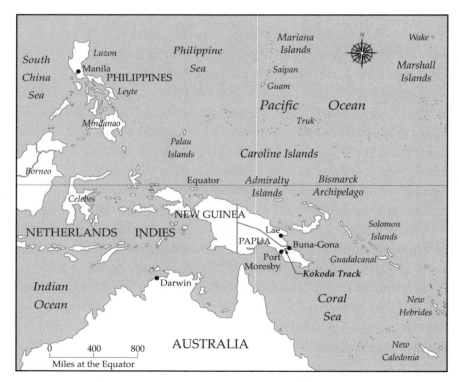

Map 4. The South and Southwest Pacific Campaign

especially in the wet months of January, February, May, and June. Malaria was hyperendemic among the local inhabitants, and the large majority of children had telltale large spleens. Every inhabitant of some villages had malaria, and the parasite accounted for nearly 20 percent of hospitalizations among Europeans new to the island.

When the Japanese landed 16,000 troops on the north coast across from Port Moresby on July 21, MacArthur was caught by surprise. Buna and the south coast were connected by the Kokoda Track, a rough footpath stretching sixty miles through the jungle and up over the Owen Stanley Range separating the north from the south coast. Maj. Gen. Tomitaro Horii planned to use the track, but he did not know it was only two feet wide in places and slimy mud almost everywhere. The track's first half rose 1,200 feet to the village of Kokoda. From there the seven-thousand-foot ascent to the top of the range was punishing, but the altitude kept it mosquito-free. Unfortunately for Horii most of his soldiers were already infected when they started the climb.

MacArthur had planned to send troops under Brig. Gen. Robert H. Van Volkenburgh to build an airfield at Buna, from which Japanese bases at Lae and Salamaua farther west on the north coast of New Guinea could be attacked. Those plans had to be changed on July 17 when Van Volkenburgh received reports that troop transports had been sighted leaving Rabaul headed toward New Guinea. Those reports verified Japanese intercepts deciphered by Navy codebreakers two months earlier that described a coming invasion. Van Volkenburgh tried to get MacArthur to dispatch troops to forestall the expected landing, but the general was busy moving his headquarters from Melbourne to Brisbane and could not be bothered.

The Australians, despite being maligned by MacArthur as nothing but city slum dwellers who would not fight, won a small but important victory at Imita Ridge on the Kokoda Track and averted a Japanese landing at Milne Bay on the eastern tip of Papua. The Kokoda campaign was, however, more a story of disease than of combat. Both sides were crippled by dysentery and beriberi, but especially by malaria.

Although malaria was rampant among Australian troops in Port Moresby, the toll was even higher among the Japanese. The initial march over the Owen Stanley Range toward Port Moresby in August was met with only limited resistance from Australian troops. The Japanese came almost within sight of Port Moresby before a lack of supplies and malaria forced them back to the north coast. They were reported to have suffered an appalling (and difficult to believe) 45 percent mortality from the disease on the Kokoda Track.[34] If the number is accurate it may have been a combination of malaria and starvation that rendered a mortality rate almost fifty times that among American forces and over twice that of the Australians.

Reliable numbers for malaria in New Guinea among the Japanese are lacking, but some idea of the prevalence can be gleaned from their experience in Rabaul. Documents captured at Munda on New Georgia give summaries of December 1942 to January 1943 and detailed data for February 1943. There were 51,382 cases of malaria in December and 79,901 in February with an admission rate of 4,086/1,000 per year, twice that of American troops. In February 20 percent of Japanese troops in Rabaul were under medical care, the vast majority for malaria.[35] If the numbers in New Guinea were similar—and they were likely worse given the conditions—the Japanese were worse off than the Allies, who were in bad shape themselves.

In October 1942, MacArthur sent three combat regiments of the 32nd Division and several Australian troops up the south end of the Kokoda Track across the Owen Stanleys to retake Buna-Gona, but the assault stalled and was almost aborted by malaria. The malaria rate in U.S. troops in Papua started at 95/1,000 per year in October and exploded to 1,672/1,000 in January. Some units saw rates as high as 3,308/1,000, and rates among Australians were reported to be four times that.[36] When the assault stalled MacArthur sent Lt. Gen. Robert Eichelberger to take command of a sick, demoralized force in which some two-hundred-man rifle companies were down to just sixty-five men.

Between October 1942 and April 1943 there were ten times as many hospital admissions for malaria as for battle casualties, and a majority of Allied divisions in the theater were incapable of effective military use. In December the rate among American troops was 600/1,000 per year; by the end of the Buna-Gona Campaign that rate peaked at 6,600/1,000.[37] New arrivals were at particular risk, and about three-quarters of the cases were virulent *falciparum*. In 1943 alone the Southwest Pacific Area reported 47,663 cases of malaria with an additional 13,320 cases of fever of unknown origin that were, in 70–80 percent of cases, malaria as well.[38] Between 1942 and 1945 in the Southwest Pacific theater there were 124,109 confirmed malaria hospitalizations.[39]

Malaria was also eating up hospital beds needed for battle casualties. Between October 1942 and April 1943 there were as many as ten times as many hospital beds occupied by malaria patients as by battle casualties in the Southwest Pacific.[40] The hospitalization rate for malaria peaked in February at 794/1,000 per year with an average hospital stay of more than fifteen days.

And the disease lingered; troops were typically ineffective for four to six months after being removed from a malarious area. Ten months after leaving New Guinea, 67 percent of the 32nd Division still had symptomatic malaria. In the Buna-Gona Campaign, the 7,679-man 32nd Division had 5,358 cases of malaria or undiagnosed fever. After leaving Papua 67 percent of its personnel still had clinical malaria, and the unit was ineffective for almost six months.[41]

MacArthur told his medical officer, Paul Russell, "Doctor this will be a long war if for every division I have facing the enemy I must count on a second division in hospital with malaria and a third division convalescing from this debilitating disease."[42] MacArthur came to the harsh realization that *Anopheles* mosquitoes were a bigger threat than Japanese bullets. So had his staff. Chief of professional services at the Office of the Surgeon General of the Army Brig. Gen. Charles C. Hillman in June 1943: "It should be realized that there is much greater danger of defeat of the American Forces in this theater by this disease alone tha[n] as a result of casualties inflicted by the [Japanese]."[43] Brig. Gen. Hugh J. Morgan, also of the Office of the Surgeon General: "The greatest threat to successful military operations in this theater is malaria. The Japanese are responsible for only 10–15% of the evacuation from the front. Malaria is responsible for over 50%. Thus, the enemy's influence upon our non-effective rate is negligible as compared to the effect of malaria." He estimated that ineffectiveness from malaria was five to ten times that from enemy fire.[44] Eichelberger: "We had to whip the Japanese before the malaria mosquito whipped us."[45]

MacArthur established the Combined Advisory Committee on Tropical Medicine, Hygiene and Sanitation in March 1943 reporting directly to his headquarters. Col. Howard F. Smith was named theater malariologist and charged with coordinating research and medical efforts against malaria in the theater. Malaria had become a priority, but it still took a great deal of time and effort to bring it under control. MacArthur's people had four major problems. Line commanders were not committed to malaria control; drugs and antimalarial supplies were low on the priority list for shipment to Australia and New Guinea; medical officers were woefully ignorant of prevention, diagnosis, and treatment of malaria; and coordinated policies for managing malaria in the U.S. Army in the Pacific did not exist.

The Army had not learned Slim's lesson from Burma. The health of troops in general and control of malaria in particular were still the responsibility of officers who had no doubt Japanese soldiers were lethal but were not at all convinced about mosquitoes. When malaria crippled a unit it was easiest to just blame the unit doctor. That was unfair for two reasons. First the combat surgeon could give advice only. Issuing orders to the troops was up to the unit commander. Second almost none of the medical officers had ever seen a case of malaria.

Col. Benjamin Baker, who had been a professor at Johns Hopkins and would later serve as MacArthur's chief consultant in medicine, admitted as much: "I didn't know anything about malaria, never heard of a case of malaria except from my father."[46] Dr. George Sharp, battalion surgeon for the 20th Infantry Regiment of the 6th Infantry Division, was frank: "I don't know what the line people thought, 'cause they were relying on us who didn't know what we were doing."[47]

To understand the Medical Corps' predicament it helps to look at what happened to that branch early in the war. In June 1939, the surgeon general headed an Army Medical Department with direct control over 9,359 officers and enlisted men and seven general and 119 station hospitals serving a garrison army of 190,000. By October 1942 there were forty-one general, eleven evacuation, and four surgical hospitals, none of which was equipped to treat tropical disease. At its peak in June 1945 the Army had 8,366,373 men and women, and the Medical Corps was four times the size the entire Army had been six years earlier. The number of Medical Department officers went from 2,181 to 142,616, and nurses increased from 672 to 54,291. Enlisted men in the department soared from 9,359 to 521,282. Not surprisingly the largest percentage increase was in administrators who went from 64 to 19,893.[48]

The Markle Foundation did supply a $170,000 grant that allowed medical schools to send one or two staff members to be trained at the Army Medical School and in tropical medicine clinics in Central America. Sixty-six of the nation's seventy-three medical schools took advantage of the funding so there was a slowly growing pipeline of trained physicians, but none had been trained when MacArthur needed them in New Guinea.

Equipment, insecticides, and drugs for malaria control were also a problem. Those supplies were tenth on the shipping priority list, well below arms, clothing, and just about everything else. Screens, mosquito nets, larvicides, repellants, and antimalarial drugs sat on docks in the United States waiting for transport. MacArthur had them moved to the top of the list.

A real problem was the total lack of anyone with expertise with insects, so mosquito control units were formed. Malaria came to the Army's attention when Caribbean bases were turned over as part of a Lend Lease trade in the fall of 1940. A unit for tropical disease control was formed as a subdivision of the Preventive Medicine division in April 1941. It was charged with collecting data on tropical disease in U.S. possessions and bases and evaluating drugs and equipment for malaria control, but it comprised only four officers. By late 1942, it was clear commanders in the Pacific Theater needed help.

A malaria control organization devoted to overseas areas was formed within the Army Medical Department in September 1942. Malaria units were divided into survey groups to assess the severity of the problem and necessary solutions and control units charged with actual mosquito management. By the beginning of October there were medical and sanitary personnel whose only responsibility was malaria. A typical unit had one or two malariologists, and survey units had an entomologist, a parasitologist, and laboratory personnel. The control units had a sanitary engineer and eleven enlisted technicians. Local labor gangs augmented by enlisted men did the hard work of draining and filling mosquito breeding sites.

Those units were deployed in the South Pacific by January 1943 and to Central Africa, China-Burma-India, the Middle East, North Africa, and the Caribbean Defense Command shortly thereafter. By July there were thirty-one malariologists either deployed or en route, virtually all of whom came from an eight-week course in tropical medicine at the Army Medical School.[49] Entomologists and parasitologists were recruited from faculty and graduate students at various universities, and sanitary engineers were drafted from local public health departments. Enlisted men were the hardest to come by since the Army would only assign recruits to malaria units. That meant sixteen or seventeen weeks of basic training followed by weeks of specialty training in malaria control before the men could be deployed.

It was a six-month process, and the Army could not wait for fully staffed units. By the summer of 1943 every unit of company size in the Pacific had at least two enlisted men and a noncommissioned officer assigned to repairing netting and screens, oiling standing water, and swatting and spraying mosquitoes. The first fully staffed control unit in the Pacific was finally deployed in February 1943 with Col. Howard F. Smith was appointed as "Theater Malariologist."

In March 1943 MacArthur set up the U.S.-Australia Combined Advisory Committee on Tropical Medicine, Hygiene and Sanitation that reported directly to his headquarters. In May Col. Paul F. Russell, chief of the Tropical Disease and Malaria Control Branch of the Preventive Medicine Division of the Office of the Surgeon General, came to Australia to meet directly with MacArthur. By June there were units throughout the area and malaria rates were dropping.

By mid-February 1944 there were 1,235 officers and men overseas in survey and control units. The Army ultimately committed to one survey and one control unit for each division or for each 20,000 deployed men. For an "important post or station," the ratio was increased to one unit per 7,500 men.[50] By the end of the war, there were 68 survey and 159 control units with 60 newly trained malariologists deployed. Had the war lasted there would have been 130 survey and 278 control units in the Pacific theater alone. The Army created a massive new specialty organization and staffed it in a matter of months.

Swatting mosquitoes and draining the pools where they bred were well enough, but the real ecological solution looked to be larvicides and chemicals to kill adult insects. An aerosol "bug bomb" was developed at a USDA laboratory in Orlando, Florida, in 1941. The bomb used pyrethrum and Freon propellant and could remove mosquitoes in 150,000 cubic feet of space, and, by March 1943, 600,000 of the "bombs" had been produced. Inventive GIs also figured out how to remove the Freon and jury rig beer refrigerators.

One of the two great advances in malaria control that came with the war was dichlorodiphenyltrichloroethane (DDT). It had first been synthesized in Vienna in 1874 by chemistry student Othnian Zeidler, but its insecticide properties were not discovered until 1939 by Paul Muller of Geiger Laboratories in Switzerland who received a Nobel Prize for the discovery. By 1940, it was being sold as Gesarol to control potato bugs and as Neocid to kill lice. Maj. A. R. W. de Jonge, a U.S. military attaché in Bern, sent samples to the United States in 1942, and the Bureau of Entomology and Plant Quarantine showed it to be effective against a range of insects including mosquitoes.

DDT had the signal advantage of lasting as much as six weeks after a single application. The War Production Board put it on the Army supply list in May 1943 and undertook a variety of experiments with airborne sprayers, some piloted by former crop dusters. Although aerial DDT spraying was effective it came too late to have significant impact on malaria in the Pacific.

Repellants were another story. Over 7,000 compounds were tested before finding dimethyl phthalate. DEET was an effective repellant, especially when mixed with Rutgers 612 and Indalone as "6-2-2," but it was oily, smelled bad, stained clothes, and, as noted previously, dissolved plastic. Besides, it sweated off and had to be constantly reapplied. The soldiers hated it. An attempt was made to issue lighter-weight long-sleeve shirts and long pants as a substitute, but the soldiers just cut off the pants and shed the shirts.

Controlling insect vectors was not the only solution. Malaria requires not only the insect but also a human host, and that is where the real success came, albeit not without difficulty.

By February 1943 MacArthur's staff had gotten serious. Shirts and long pants were mandated between sundown and sunrise although enforcement was spotty. Mosquito bars and repellants were issued to every man, but their use was spotty as well. Anything containing standing water within one thousand yards of sleeping quarters was to be oiled or drained, including cans, bottles, coconut shells, and tire tracks. More to the point, commanding officers of all grades were responsible for implementing sanitary regulations. In Australia aborigines with malaria were rounded up and held in compounds away from mosquito breeding areas.

But cleaning up the environment, removing local carriers, and covering up the soldiers were not what brought malaria under control. That took drugs, but to be effective the drugs had to be taken. Atabrine and quinine were administered under direct observation in all hyperendemic areas. Between November 1942 and the following April the standard regimen for acute disease was a fifteen-day course with quinine, Atabrine, and Plasmochin given sequentially (QAP therapy). The quinine was first because low doses of Atabrine were slow to take effect, and malaria had a distressing tendency to recur just after Atabrine was started.

Like quinine, Atabrine taken continuously and in sufficient doses while in a malarious area prevented the disease. One or the other was supposed to be started seven days before troops left Australia and continued until the soldiers withdrew to malaria-free bases. The problem was getting the men to take the drug, and that led to "Atabrine formations." Combat units were called out by roster and lined up with men three feet apart holding cups to which half inch of water was added from a lyster bag. The cup was held in the left hand while an Atabrine pill was placed in the right. Without closing his hand the soldier tossed the pill into his mouth, emptied the cup, and put it upside down on a table. He then moved forward three feet where his name and rank were checked against the unit roster before he went to an at-ease formation and waited five minutes to make sure he did not spit the pill out. That was all very well when the men were on base, but the regimen fell apart when the units went into combat.

Although *falciparum* was often cured if Atabrine was continued for four weeks after the last symptom, *vivax* hid in the liver. It resurfaced when the drugs were stopped, and *vivax* was eventually more than six times as frequent as *falciparum*. If drugs were stopped after the acute episode at least half of the cases recurred in the first month. Recurrence proved as big a problem as prevention.

Without an accepted standard of dose and frequency, every unit surgeon became a de facto researcher, but the "experiments" were disorganized, unrecorded, and devoid of useful information. Real experiments were necessary, and a series of them were started on soldiers in Australia and on "volunteers" in the United States.

Brigadier N. Hamilton Fairley tried various Atabrine doses on Australian soldiers, and by early 1943 he demonstrated that the drug could cure *falciparum* if given long enough and in high enough doses and would suppress *vivax* as long as it was continued.[51] The Land Headquarters (LHQ) research unit at Cairns had a sixty-bed mosquito-proof ward staffed with physicians, pathologists, and entomologists experienced with malaria. Soldiers were subject to bites from infected mosquitoes or direct injection of parasites after which various regimens of quinine, atabrine, and sulfonamides were tried.[52]

Atabrine at a dose of two hundred milligrams a day starting two months before entering a malarious area and continued for two more months after leaving along with a maintenance suppressive dose of one hundred milligrams a day while exposed proved effective. The high predeployment dose assumed that men would stop taking the drug as soon as they were in the field. The Americans did similar experiments at Milne Bay and Catton, Queensland, and came to the same conclusion. The regimen became standard throughout the Pacific.[53]

Australian malaria experiments were not only on soldiers. Melbourne's *The Age* and the *Sydney Morning Herald* reported that Italian and German internees and Jewish refugees transferred from Britain were deliberately infected as subjects in drug trials.[54]

The Sixth U.S. Army Training Center was established "to receive from combat units personnel infected with malaria and to prepare them physically and mentally for further combat duty."[55] Seven programs were designed to test different Atabrine doses, and the men were followed for splenomegaly, changes in hemoglobin, weight loss, abdominal pain, diarrhea, vomiting, fever, hypertension, albuminuria, skin discoloration, and parasites on blood smear. Most importantly, Atabrine blood levels were monitored. Less than 1 percent of the men had "unfavorable reactions" although what constituted unfavorable is not clear. Even when suppressive doses were continued over long periods the disease regularly recurred two to four weeks after Atabrine was stopped. Atabrine suppressed *vivax* but did not cure it, and the drug was basically gone from the blood after four days, so it had to be given at least twice a week and for long periods.

Another series of experiments proved that men on suppression could endure hard exercise for up to eighty hours a week without ill effects. Once again the drug was intended to keep men in combat not cure them.

In the United States the Office of Scientific Research and Development contracted with the National Research Council to study malaria. The council combined with the Army, the Navy, and the U.S. Public Health Service to coordinate studies of Atabrine and repellants. Vannevar Bush headed the Office of Scientific Research and Development including a seven-member Committee on Medical Research comprising mostly academicians convinced that the vicissitudes of war justified the risk of human experimentation. The committee was, however, hesitant to experiment on soldiers; they preferred conscientious objectors or prisoners.

The Malaria Research Program was started in 1944 at the federal penitentiary in Atlanta, at the New Jersey State Reformatory, at the U.S. Army Disciplinary Barracks in Green Haven, New York, and at the Stateville Penitentiary thirty miles outside Chicago. Prisoners were offered better living conditions, minimal pay (typically $20 for drug toxicity studies and $100 for getting malaria), and the suggestion of earlier parole. They were told that participation in the experiments was a way for patriotic prisoners to contribute to the war effort. They were told they would help find drugs that were safe for "our fighting men" including finding how high a dose of an antimalarial "could be tolerated by the human system." Several hundred men were enlisted to serve as "human test tubes."[56] When principal investigator Alf Sven Alving of the University of Chicago told prospective volunteers that malaria was the biggest medical problem in the Pacific and was costing the Army more men than Japanese bullets, he had no difficulty getting experimental subjects.

The most extensive program was at Stateville beginning in 1944. The program continued into the Vietnam War years during which thousands of prisoners were infected with malaria. Some were experimental subjects, but others just served as reservoirs for parasites to be used in later studies—human malaria banks. *Falciparum* was occasionally used but most often the pathogen was the Chesson strain of *vivax*. That strain was particularly virulent causing disease of quicker onset and greater severity so the experiments could be shorter. Some subjects were infected with mosquito bites; others were infected by implanting mosquito salivary glands under their skin.[57]

> Prisoners competed to participate, and each signed a blanket waiver: I assume the risks of this experiment and I absolve the University of Chicago and all the technicians and researchers who take part in the experiment, as well as the government of Illinois, the directory of the State penitentiary and every other official, even as concerns my heirs and representatives of any responsibility.[58]

The inmates were considered in the odd legal condition of *homine sacres*—a life that might be taken without the commission of homicide. They were, however, given valuable consideration for their participation. Governor Adlai Stevenson commuted or paroled 317 of the volunteers including twenty-four convicted of homicide or rape.[59]

For first "bite day" on March 8 mosquitoes were fed on patients from Manteno State Hospital for the Insane who had been deliberately infected with *vivax* malaria as a treatment for syphilitic dementia.[60] After infection the Stateville volunteers were not given antimalarials until they had a fever of at least 102° and often as high as 106°.

The most famous participant was Nathan Leopold who, with his partner and probable lover Richard Loeb, had kidnapped and murdered fourteen-year-old Bobby Frank on a lark while both were students at the University of Chicago. In their sensational trial, Leopold, defended by Clarence Darrow, pled guilty and was spared the death penalty. While serving a sentence of life plus ninety-nine years, he worked as a researcher, laboratory technician, and experimental volunteer in the malaria experiments.[61] Leopold later used that participation in a successful parole application.

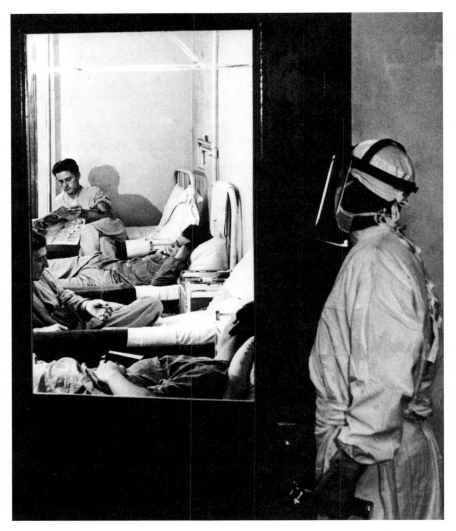

Federal prisoners at the U.S. penitentiary in Seagonville, Texas, participating in malaria experiments in the 1940s. *National Library of Medicine*

There were also attempts to develop a malaria vaccine including experiments in which 2 to 3 billion dead *vivax* organisms were injected into prisoners some of whom may have been Italian and German prisoners of war.[62]

Prisoners were better experimental subjects than soldiers. They were cheap, available, and under stringent control—as close to laboratory animals as possible. The ethics of using prisoners for medical experiments are complicated by the serious question about whether an inmate is capable of giving voluntary, uncoerced consent, but it was a quick way to get necessary information.

Australians and Americans were not the only ones using prisoners in malaria experiments. Dr. Klaus Schilling studied pyramidon, aspirin, quinine, and Atabrine in 1,200 German concentration camp inmates. He used high and sometimes lethal doses on inmates of mental asylums in Italy and later at Dachau. Similar experiments were done by Professor Gerhard Rose on Russian prisoners of war and at a psychiatric clinic in Thuringia. Schilling was executed in 1946 and Rose was given a life sentence, although for typhus experiments rather than those on malaria. Defense lawyers at Nuremberg unsuccessfully cited the Stateville malaria experiments on behalf of their clients.

In any event, when the correct dose and schedule for Atabrine were worked out the results were stunning. After mid-1943 malaria no longer seriously impacted military operations in the Southwest Pacific Area of Operations. In January 1943, the malaria attack rate at Milne Bay was 3,308/1,000 per year. In January 1944 it was 30.7/1,000. In the whole Southwest Area, the attack rate in February 1943 was 794/1,000 per year. A year later it was 179/1,000, and it was less than 50/1,000 by May. An estimated 9,600 hospital beds were freed for other uses.[63]

The Australians did not fare as well. They had more men deployed in the jungle, but they also had more difficulty getting their men to take Atabrine. At the peak there were areas with an attack rate of 4,840/1,000 per year among Australian soldiers, most of which were relapses after the drug was stopped. Doubling the dose and more rigid enforcement of malaria discipline brought the rate down to 740/1,000 per year by December, and it continued to drop thereafter.[64]

The Australians were particularly worried that troops returning from malarious areas would precipitate an epidemic in parts of Queensland known to harbor *Anopheles*. After November 1942, troops returning from New Guinea and Guadalcanal were excluded from Australia north of 19°S until they had been proven malaria-free for six months and were on suppressive medications. Those rules applied to American troops as well and were kept in place until the war ended even though there was never a domestic malaria outbreak in Australia.[65] In 1942, there were only twelve cases of malaria in all of Australia.[66]

The Australians took Gona on December 9, 1942, and Buna fell on January 2. Sanananda fell in January 22, and the north coast of Papua was secured. Under Operation Cartwheel MacArthur was to move west along the northern coast of New Guinea. The Japanese attempted to bring two fresh divisions from Rabaul under Lieutenant General Adachi Hatuzo, but most of those troops were lost in the Battle of the Bismarck Sea before they got to New Guinea.

By late spring 40 percent of the Japanese troops still in New Guinea were malnourished and had malaria. The disease the Americans and Australians were well on the way to controlling still ravaged the Japanese, and they were unable to withstand the assault that summer by better-armed, better-supplied, and healthier Allied troops. New Guinea was retaken, and attention was turned to the Philippines.

Malaria control, partially from mosquito control but mostly due to Atabrine, made MacArthur's campaign a success. By the time he returned to the Philippines MacArthur reported that the disease was "reduced to secondary importance as a cause of disablement and no longer deserved serious consideration in planning tactical operations."[67]

The Solomons

But we need to take a step back. At the same time MacArthur was taking New Guinea from the Japanese and malaria, the enemy and the parasite were being fought farther east in the South Pacific.

The compromise strategy in which MacArthur and Nimitz would each command his own area was built around a three-task strategy. Task 1 was an attack on the island of Tulagi by Ghormley and the amphibious 1st Marine Division. Since those were Nimitz's troops, his boundary with MacArthur's area was shifted west by one degree. Task 2 had two parts. MacArthur was to secure New Guinea while the Marines and supplemental Army units moved up the Solomon Islands. The final task brought the two forces together to attack the huge Japanese base at Rabaul.

The Americans landed unopposed one thousand miles east of Australia on Efate on April 8 and on Espiritu Santo to the northwest on May 4.

Airstrips that could be used to attack the Japanese in the Solomons were built on both islands. It was 1,550 miles from Efate to Emirau where the South Pacific campaign finally ended on March 20, 1944, after the construction of eleven military bases on 24,000 square miles of malarious islands.

Marines arrived on Efate in the New Hebrides on April 8, 1942, but they made no attempt to control mosquitoes and did not take suppressive drugs. The malaria attack rate soared to 2,632/1,000 per year.[68] That was just a foretaste of what was to come. Before the war was over malaria caused five times as many casualties as combat, and the worst of it was on Guadalcanal.[69]

Operation Watchtower—the attack on the Solomons—was pushed up to the first week of August 1942 when Nimitz learned the Japanese were building an airfield on Guadalcanal and a seaplane base at nearby Tulagi, either of which would threaten the sea lanes connecting Australia to North America. Forces for an amphibious attack collected in Fiji along with seventy-six warships under Vice Adm. Frank Jack Fletcher who was fresh from victories at Coral Sea and Midway. The force had three of the Navy's four remaining aircraft carriers, its brand-new battleship, and a division of cruisers from the Royal Australian Navy. Rear Adm. Richmond Kelly Turner commanded Amphibious Force South Pacific—the ships carrying the 1st Marine Division—a regiment from the 2nd Marine Division, and a smattering of other units.

The operation started smoothly. Tulagi and the small adjoining islands of Gavutu and Tanambogo fell quickly, and the airfield at Guadalcanal was in American hands by August 8. The rest of the island was not. That took five more agonizing months.

Fletcher, jealously protective of his carriers, pulled them out within four days of the landing on Guadalcanal leaving the Marines with a four-day supply of ammunition and enough food for two meals a day. The Marines were also unprotected from a still formidable Japanese fleet. The partially completed airstrip was renamed Henderson Field and rushed to completion so the force could at least be resupplied by air.

Meanwhile the Japanese had concentrated their forces on New Guinea assuming that they could retake Guadalcanal whenever they got around to it. They did send a small number of troops from Rabaul in a desultory attempt to capture the island but suffered a resounding defeat at the Ilu River. That was just the beginning of a two-month effort by each side to put troops on the island and supply them. The Americans controlled the skies during the day, but the Japanese owned the sea around Guadalcanal after dark. Rear Admiral Raizo Tanaka's Tokyo Express shipped in troops and supplies every night. Guadalcanal was a series of epic naval battles and constant air combat while troops on the island fought each other, the jungle, and mosquitoes.

Guadalcanal, the largest of the Solomon Islands, is 2,047 square miles of volcanic rock with interior mountains rising over 7,500 feet. The mountainsides are covered with dense rainforest crisscrossed with fast-running streams. The rainforests were too thick for bivouacking, were barely passable, and were not a serious malaria risk. But the base of the mountains was covered with coconut, cacao, and coffee plantations whose rutted tracks and fields collected water and bred mosquitoes. Along the northwest coast there were flat plains with grass up to six feet high and mangrove swamps saturated by as much as one hundred inches of rain a year. That and an average year-round temperature of 80°F made malaria hyperendemic.

When the Marines landed in August—the dry season—mosquitoes were relatively uncommon, and malaria was infrequent. "No attempt was made at first to carry out individual protective measures, to enforce suppressive medication, or to combat mosquitoes."[70] The resulting laxness in "malaria discipline" cost the marines dearly when the rains came and mosquitoes hatched.[71]

Of the 100,000 cases of malaria in U.S. forces in the South Pacific, 60,000 were on Guadalcanal.[72] As we have seen repeatedly, epidemic disease always takes second place to the drama of combat. One of the more comprehensive descriptions of the Guadalcanal campaign devotes more print to the arrival of turkey dinners for the Marines than to malaria.[73]

Falciparum was twice as common as *vivax* when the Marines first landed, but as *falciparum* was treated it was gradually replaced by recurrent *vivax*, and by January 1944 *vivax* was twenty times as common. Malaria was present in 91 percent of Guadalcanal's children under five, and 73 percent of all children on the island had enlarged spleens.[74] They were an inexhaustible reservoir of disease.

Malaria broke out in the 1st Marine Division in August with nine hundred cases. In September there were 1,724, in October 2,630, and in mid-December the division had 8,500 men hospitalized with malaria. Within nine months, 80 percent of the division had been hospitalized at least once for malaria. The Department of the Navy said almost every man who served between August 7, 1942, and February 9, 1943, had malaria.[75] And many had it more than once. In February, while adherence to malaria discipline was negligible, the reported incidence peaked at 1,781/1,000 per year for all forces on the island.[76] The attack rate was almost certainly much higher since Maj. Gen. Alexander Vandergrift ordered that no one with a temperature less than 103°F be excused from duty.[77]

The one bright spot for the Marines was that the Japanese suffered even more. As in New Guinea there are few exact records of the malaria incidence among the Japanese, but what we have describes a truly dire situation. There were few Japanese prisoners taken, but virtually all who were captured had malaria. There is some data on the rate among Japanese in the Solomons in February 1943. That attack rate was recorded as 1,637/1,000/ year, but data from Rabaul in 1943 (2,503/1,000/year) suggests that was an underestimate.[78] Japanese troops had limited supplies of larvicide, nets, repellants, and antimalarial drugs. The disease was also aggravated by the high incidence of malnourishment and vitamin B-1 deficiency (beriberi) in the Imperial Army. Of roughly 33,600 Japanese troops sent to Guadalcanal, 19,200 (65 percent) died. For every soldier who died in combat two died of disease. Japan lost Guadalcanal to malnutrition and malaria.

At any given time the Empire's troops were functioning at one-third to one-fifth strength, but it was not all good news for the Americans. Along with infected local inhabitants the Japanese troops were a reservoir. *Anopheles* can easily fly a mile and a half, and infected Japanese were regularly closer than that. Their bullets might not hit an American soldier, but their mosquitoes certainly did.

As MacArthur had in New Guinea, Adm. William F. Halsey, newly in command of the South Pacific Area (SOPAC), realized he had a serious problem. By November 1942, he had deployed malaria control units and had ordered every line commander to cooperate with the units' suggestions and to consult with them before constructing camps and airfields.

"We are here to fight Japs, not mosquitoes" was no longer an acceptable attitude among the officers, but the men had to be convinced. Half the draftees in World War II were high school graduates, and 10 percent had been in college; they have been justifiably called the best-educated enlisted force in history, but once in the military they were taught by Walt Disney and Dr. Seuss. The War Department produced fifteen antimalaria posters, three cartoon motion pictures, and a recording, and distributed 25,000 copies of each.[79] Warner Brothers and Disney competed to produce a series of educational cartoons. The contract went to Warner Brothers because Disney refused to surrender rights to the characters. Frank Capra, head of the Information and Education Division of

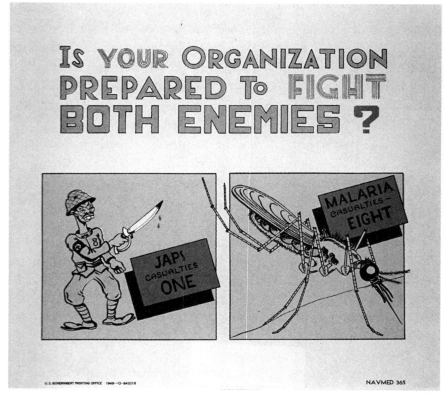

A U.S. government poster from 1945, the final year of World War II. It was difficult to convince soldiers in the Pacific Theater that mosquitoes were as dangerous as the Japanese. *National Library of Medicine*

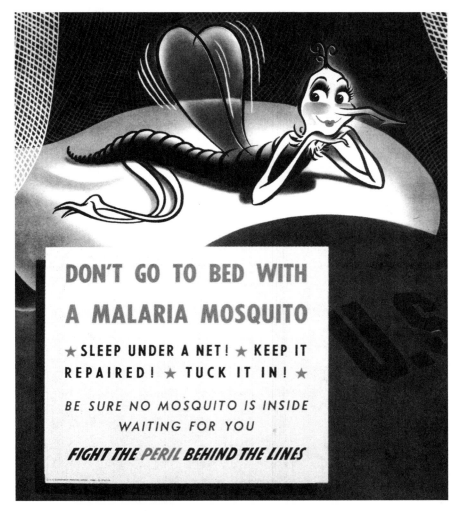

A U.S. government poster from 1944. Sex was used as well as patriotism to encourage use of mosquito nets. *National Library of Medicine*

the U.S. Army, was in charge of the education program. Theodore Geisel (Dr. Seuss) led the animation branch that produced the Private Snafu series of three-minute training pieces between 1943 and 1946. Private Snafu was a weak, lazy, incompetent soldier with a Brooklyn accent provided by Mel Blanc. He resisted long sleeves, mosquito nets, repellants, and Atabrine, and invariably came to a bad end. His postmortem said, "This program has come to you through the courtesy of my sponsors, the United States Army, distributors of GI repellant, mosquito nets, Atabrine tablets, and good old-fashioned horse sense. Gee, I wish to hell I'd used them."[80] Although they missed out on the contract to supply regular content, Disney did produce *The Winged Scourge*, a longer feature using Snow White's seven dwarves to hang nets and drain standing water while dodging giant mosquitoes.

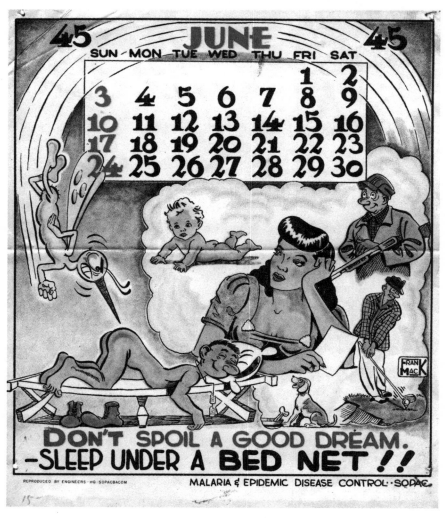

A U.S. Army cartoon from 1945 promoting the use of bed nets to help prevent malaria from mosquito bites. *National Library of Medicine*

There were malaria control signs on arrival docks that featured scantily clad women and Burma Shave–style serial signs on the roadways. Armed Forces Radio aired repeated reminders interspersed with fifteen minutes of music in the "Atabrine Cocktail Hour" from the "Fungus festooned fern room" in downtown Guadalcanal. Some propaganda bordered on the macabre. The entrance to the 363rd Station Hospital had a sign flanked by two human skulls that read "These Men Didn't Take Their Atabrine."

The Americans were not the only ones dispensing malaria propaganda. Tokyo Rose broadcast warnings that Atabrine caused permanent liver damage and would make a soldier who took it useless to any young native lady he happened to encounter. Besides, he would be sterile when he went home.

Although rumors of liver damage, sterility, and infertility were untrue, Atabrine was not without problems, most of which were related to doses that were either too small or too large. When it was initially used on Guadalcanal at a dose of two hundred milligrams per day—twice what was eventually settled on—Atabrine caused many Marines (including commanding officer Maj. Gen. Alexander M. Patch) diarrhea and nausea. When the dose was decreased to fifty milligrams per day the gastrointestinal side effects stopped, but the drug was ineffective. It took time to arrive at one hundred milligrams per day, which prevented malaria and had few side effects.

Perhaps the worst Atabrine mistake was stopping the drug as soon as troops left malarious areas. The assumption was that malaria might recur, but the men would have an episode of illness, build their immunity, and be ready to return to combat. That was disastrously wrong. The 147th Infantry Regiment had sporadically taken Atabrine while on Guadalcanal and had an attack rate of 1,000 cases/1,000 men/year while on the island. When the regiment went to Samoa the drug was abruptly stopped. In the next five months the rate increased to 3,000/1,000/year, and in some groups was an astronomical 14,000/1,000. When Atabrine was restarted the rate dropped to 100/1,000.[81]

The Americal Division had a similar experience. They arrived on Guadalcanal in echelons between October and December 1942 and rarely took Atabrine. Their malaria rate spiked to 1,358/1,000. In March the division went to Fiji and its soldiers were treated with Atabrine and Plasmochin until June when the drugs were stopped. The rate rocketed to 3,760/1,000/year by August.[82] Atabrine was restarted in November, and the rate dropped to 43/1,000 by January.[83] Of the 15,000 men who went to Fiji from Guadalcanal there were 75,000 malaria attacks within a year of stopping suppression.[84] The 1st Marine Division and the 32nd Army Division were unable to return to combat for six months after withdrawal from Guadalcanal and New Guinea respectively.[85]

But when Atabrine was taken and continued the results were stunning. On Efate, the attack rate in April 1942 was 2,678/1,000/year. In July, 400 mg a week (a low dose) of Atabrine was started. In August there were 209 cases, and in September there were 144. To remove the human reservoir, native laborers were given Atabrine as well. When the rate dropped the drug was stopped in September. There was an immediate spike, and Atabrine was

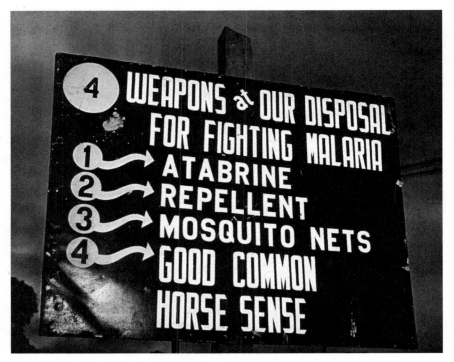

The U.S. Army finally got serious about malaria after the disease almost cost the U.S. and Australian armies New Guinea during World War II. *National Library of Medicine*

restarted in November. By July 1943 the attack rate was down to 128/1,000, sixty-two of which were recurrences.

Most of the malaria on Guadalcanal was diagnosed between October and August when there was no mosquito control and little or no Atabrine. In October 1942 the attack rate was 1,664/1000. In November, it rose to 1,781. By August 1943 the malaria control program was fully operational, and the rate was 263/1,000. By June 1945 there were only six new cases/1,000 personnel.[86] When Bougainville was taken fewer than 1 percent of the force had malaria.[87]

The Americal Division was so devastated by malaria and the "demalariazation" fiasco that there was serious question about its ever returning to combat. The division was placed on suppressive Atabrine in November. By January the attack rate was 43/1,000/year, and malaria was no longer a problem.[88] The malaria control units were reassigned to dengue, Tsutsugamushi fever, and filariasis.

The Mediterranean

The Pacific was not the only theater where malaria was a problem. The Italians and Germans and the British had pushed each other thousands of miles back and forth across North Africa in 1942 before General Erwin Rommel's defeat at El Alamein in October followed by a two-thousand-mile retreat to Tunisia during which 40,000 men—mostly Italians—were taken prisoner. In November and December German Chancellor Adolf Hitler sent 50,000 German troops and 18,000 Italians (later augmented by 100,000 Germans and 10,000 Italians) to reinforce Rommel.

Great Britain and the United States had agreed to invade North Africa, although the Americans suspected the operation was mostly to protect the Suez Canal and access to India. Resources stretched by the contemporaneous Guadalcanal campaign made a European invasion difficult, so Gen. George C. Marshall agreed to a combined North African operation commanded by Maj. Gen. Dwight D. Eisenhower. Beginning November 7, British and American forces under Maj. Gen. George S. Patton landed in Morocco and attacked Oran while a separate British force landed at Algiers.

The campaign was not without difficulty, especially for the inexperienced Americans, but Tunis fell May 13, 1943. A total of 275,000 Axis troops were captured, the vast majority of whom were Italians who represented the bulk of that country's remaining army. Most of the Germans escaped to Italy.

When Marshall arrived in Morocco for the Casablanca Conference January 14, 1943, he stepped off the plane wearing mosquito gloves, boots, and a hat with a mosquito net veil. He was met by soldiers wearing shorts and short sleeves; despite what Marshall had been told, malaria was not a problem in Morocco. That was not true of the rest of North Africa, and it was certainly not the case for Sicily and Southern Italy where the next invasion was to take place.

Operation Husky began July 9–10 with a combined amphibious invasion and air attack on Sicily. Hitler, deceived by fake plans planted on a corpse that was allowed to wash up in Italy, believed the invasion would be in Sardinia, possibly Corsica, or even Greece, but not Sicily. The island was left with ten substandard Italian divisions and two German divisions later reinforced by five more. Gen. Bernard Montgomery's advance up eastern Sicily encountered most of the resistance while Patton's advance on the west went largely unopposed. The Allies entered Messina on the north coast on August 17, by which time the Germans had already evacuated to the Italian mainland.

On July 25 the Fascist Grand Council requested that Benito Mussolini resign the office of prime minister. He was subsequently arrested by King Victor Emmanuel and replaced with Marshal Pietro Badoglio who initiated surrender discussions with the Allies. On September 3, the same day Montgomery's Eighth Army crossed the Straits of Messina and took Reggio Calabria, Italy unconditionally surrendered.

Hitler then launched Operation Alarich and took Northern Italy using troops evacuated from Sicily and men moved from France and the Russian front. The Germans occupied Rome and Generalfeldmarschall Albert Kesselring deployed the Tenth Army in the south to counter an expected Allied landing at Salerno. Rommel was sent to Milan and Turin to control the remains of the Italian Army and unruly civilians. The Germans rescued Mussolini on September 16 and established the puppet Italian Social Republic in the north.

Steep mountains running the length of the Italian peninsula forced highways up against the two coasts and provided multiple lines of natural defense against the Allied advance. The Allied landing at Salerno was well protected from the air and met no real resistance until the Germans counterattacked and nearly pushed them into the sea. More Allied troops landed at Taranto September 9, and Kesselring pulled back to his first line of defense.

Naples fell to the British October 1, but Kesselring was able to concentrate troops on the Mediterranean and Adriatic coasts and established his "Winter Position" along the Gustav Line anchored by the fortress abbey at Monte Cassino. On January 22 U.S. and British troops landed south of Rome at Anzio behind the Gustav Line. They stalled there until Maj. Gen. Lucien Truscott took command on February 23. Monte Cassino was attacked three times between February 12 and May 17 before the stronghold finally fell to Polish forces allowing Truscott to break out from Anzio. Kesselring retreated 150 miles north to the Gothic Line without opposition while Gen. Mark Clark marched into the open city of Rome on June 4. The Gothic Line held until May 2, 1945, five days before the Nazi surrender.

Malaria was endemic in Morocco, Algeria, and Tunisia but hyperendemic in Sicily and southern Italy. The primary reservoirs of disease were local Arabs, Italian prisoners of war, and Yugoslav laborers brought by the Italians. Over one thousand men with malaria were left in North Africa when Operation Husky was launched, but it was not long before cases broke out in Sicily.[89] The first was July 23, and by early August there were 8,500 in the Seventh Army and almost 12,000 in the Eighth Army. II Corps saw attack rates as high as 1,700/1,000/year some weeks.[90] Fever of unknown origin rates were even higher and the majority of those were probably malaria.

Malaria control and survey units had been available in North Africa, but they were left behind when Sicily was invaded. In truth, they would probably not have been of much use since the Americans moved around the island too quickly for mosquito control to be effective. Between July 9 and September 10, 1943, there were 21,482 hospitalizations for malaria in Sicily compared to 17,375 battle casualties. Since most of those were *vivax*, many would recur in the spring of 1944 at Anzio and Monte Cassino.[91]

Suppressive Atabrine for U.S. troops had started April 22, 1943, but a "well nigh incredible wave of incapacitating toxic episodes" were reported.[92]

The main complaints were nausea, vomiting, and diarrhea, all in unlikely frequency and five times more common in rear areas than on the front line. The troops were generally aware that malaria would not kill them, but the disease was a free pass to the hospital. German propaganda amplified that; why not stop the drugs and get a lifesaving case of malaria? "By the way, why sleep under that sticky, narrow mosquito net? Fresh air and no head-ache is the richt [*sic*] for summer; you're tired enough to sleep even without those few mosquitoes—a real he-man (emended to "regular guy") won't fuss much about them anyway. . . . And then, why do they request you to swallow those dam [*sic*] pills every day? . . . They taste awfully and they do upset your stomach. However, that is not the worst of it. Man's best strength is weakened by them. So let a nice girl cross your way and the only pleasure war sometimes offers is gone and she laughs at you."[93]

Complaints about presumed side effects did lead to an adjustment of the dosage schedule from two hundred milligrams twice a week to one hundred milligrams four times a week. As DDT became available some medical officers actively discouraged Atabrine use. Truscott disagreed. In April he sent two thousand troops of VI Corps to antimalarial training and ordered roster-supervised administration of Atabrine in addition to mosquito control. For whatever reason, the incidence of adverse reactions to Atabrine dropped to under 1 percent after Atabrine became mandatory August 14, 1943.

Italy did see the widest use of anti-mosquito spraying in the war. DDT was first tested there in August 1943 and was subsequently used in communities near Naples in 1944 after it was recognized the drug left residua that were effective for weeks after application. Between DDT and Atabrine malaria was controlled, and unlike in the Pacific never threatened success in the theater.

There was one final issue. *Vivax* malaria recurs when suppressive Atabrine is stopped and the men would eventually be going home, some to areas highly susceptible to malaria. That was the fear that led Australia to keep soldiers coming back from New Guinea isolated in the remote north of the country. In the United States thirteen states along the Gulf and Atlantic coasts and in the Mississippi valley had endemic malaria exacerbated by returning soldiers. In the early 1940s there were roughly 70,000 malaria

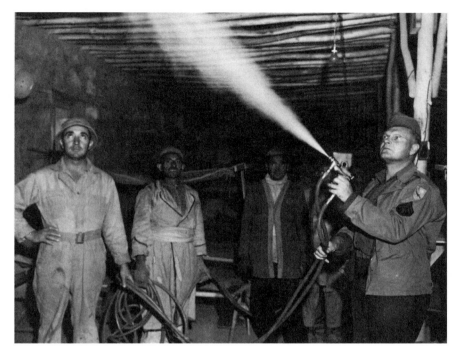

A U.S. Army photo from 1944. Spraying enlisted men's quarters with DDT was a late addition to mosquito control. *National Library of Medicine*

cases a year, a number that dropped to around 4,000 by 1950. There was even a spike where malaria was not endemic. In 1942, the non-malarious states had 656 cases; in 1943 there were 13,618.[94] There would not be a similar case rate until the Vietnam War.

Malaria nearly stole a victory from United States in the Pacific and may have cost the Japanese one. Even though other events drove the outcome in the Mediterranean, malaria caused more casualties than enemy weapons. And the means to prevent it was available from the very beginning.

CONCLUSION

After World War II

Epidemic infections continued after World War II but never in the numbers seen in the South Pacific and the Mediterranean. Cholera, typhus, filariasis, and Japanese B encephalitis were all endemic in Korea where the routine use of human feces as plant fertilizer posed a constant risk. There was a smallpox epidemic among Korean civilians in 1945–46, but 3 million doses of vaccine dispensed in the first winter of American occupation followed by an additional 18 million doses the second winter kept the disease in check, and there were only forty-four cases among U.S. soldiers.[1] A 1946 cholera epidemic caused eight thousand to ten thousand civilian deaths, but sanitary measures and an effective vaccine controlled the outbreak before American forces were affected. As many as 8 percent of Korean school children harbored malaria parasites, and antimalarial drugs were in short supply, but vigorous mosquito control thwarted that disease as well. The peak malaria incidence in the American military was 29 cases/1,000 men/year and rapidly decreased when U.S. forces broke free from the Pusan perimeter in 1950. Chloroquine, DDT, and cold weather reduced that to near zero when winter came. The incidence of dysentery went up during the Pusan concentration as well, reaching a maximum of 138.9 admissions/1,000 soldiers/year in August 1950. Korean Hemorrhagic Fever, a disease now known to be caused by rodent-borne hantavirus, was new to the Army Medical Service. Although there was no effective treatment for the disease, only about five hundred to nine hundred cases a year were hospitalized in Korea, and the mortality rate was less than 10 percent.[2]

One reason for the unusually effective control of contagion in Korea may have been because the conflict followed hard on the heels of World War II. Many of the senior medical officers in Korea had military experience and were able to teach junior officers the essentials of prevention and treatment of infectious diseases. In addition, medical supplies and drugs were flown in almost without limit from the United States, military medical research was active and well-funded, and there was a variety of new antimicrobial drugs and vaccines.

Not surprisingly, mosquito-borne diseases were relatively common in Vietnam. Dengue, characterized by leukopenia, a maculopapular rash, severe headache, and protracted recovery, had been a problem in Asia and the Pacific since the Spanish-American War. There was a dengue epidemic at Fort William McKinley outside Manila in 1906, and the incidence among American troops in the Philippines between 1902 and 1924 averaged 101/1,000/year. An estimated 40 percent of new arrivals got dengue in their first year in the islands. An epidemic in Queensland and the Northern Territories of Australia affected an estimated 80 percent of American troops stationed there in 1942, and dengue was second only to malaria in military importance in the South and Southwest Pacific areas during World War II. Still, the disease caused few deaths and was significant mostly for lost service time. That was true in Vietnam as well. Diagnosis of dengue in Vietnam was inconsistent, but a significant number of the 225,000 days lost to fevers of unknown origin were probably from that disease. Dengue also occurred in limited numbers in American troops in Somalia in 1992–93 and in Haiti in 1994.

Malaria was the most significant infectious disease during the Vietnam War. *Falciparum* strains resistant to chloroquine were identified in 1962, and primaquine was added to the drug regimen for the disease. Resistant cases continued to occur, and in November 1965 almost 110 of every 1,000 active soldiers were unable to report for duty during the six to eight weeks it took to recover. The rate decreased after 1966 when helicopter spraying of insecticides increased, personal protection including repellants and mosquito nets were required, and the anti-leprosy drug diaminodiphenylsulfone (dapsone) was added to the chloroquine-primaquine regimen.[3] The Army also embarked on the largest research program in its history, awarding more than two hundred grants worth in excess of $10 million to screen more than 130,000 potential drugs.

Diarrhea, dysentery, and hepatitis were also problematic in Vietnam, with shigellosis being particularly common and amebiasis being especially severe. Sanitary engineers and trained sanitarians were deployed throughout Southeast Asia, and the gastrointestinal infections were largely controlled. Prophylactic gamma globulin was given to prevent hepatitis, and vaccinations against yellow fever, typhus, polio, diphtheria-tetanus, typhoid, and cholera were routine. Although infectious diseases were not uncommon in Southeast Asia, improved sanitary measures, better drugs, and new vaccines kept them from reaching the military significance of former wars.

EPIDEMICS AND FUTURE CONFLICT

Counterfactual history is a perilous exercise, but outcomes in the episodes we have looked at might very well have been different had the epidemics not turned out as they did.

Gates' army was incapacitated after the withdrawal from Canada, and without control of smallpox it would have been unlikely to defeat Burgoyne's British forces. An American defeat at Saratoga would have separated New England from the rest of the colonies, and France might well have stayed out of the war.

It is hard to assess the net effect of epidemics on the Civil War since both sides suffered, but McClellan believed he would have defeated the Confederates in the Peninsular Campaign with fewer men than he lost to typhoid. Capturing Richmond might have shortened the war by two years.

Had yellow fever persisted in Cuba, the United States might well have done what every other colonizing power except Spain had done. Fear of yellow fever led to the Round Robin letter and the precipitous withdrawal of American troops. The administrative force left behind might have left as well if there had been an outbreak. Had the U.S. Army abandoned the island the Panama Canal would probably not have been dug when it was.

Had the Army not been so anxious to get men out of Fort Riley and the other cantonments, influenza might not have spread to Europe. Without influenza the Ludendorff Offensive might have resulted in a French defeat and British withdrawal from the war.

MacArthur said his army could not function with the incidence of malaria it was suffering. Without Atabrine New Guinea and Guadalcanal might well have remained in Japanese hands. Australia might have been cut off and Japan might have settled in for a long Pacific occupation.

The current pandemic has not had significant military consequences beyond confining combat ships to port, but that is largely because there were no major conflicts during the early months of COVID-19. It is not unlikely that a future war will coincide with a pandemic and have its outcome affected, if not determined, by a disease, and we will probably still have the same four tools to combat it.

Quarantine is the least effective and conflicts with warfare's need to collect and move masses of humans. The influenza epidemic is the starkest example of what happens when the infected are mixed with the susceptible. COVID-19 has provided grim evidence of quarantine's limitations. Its effect on the Ukrainian War is, as yet, unknown, although there does not seem to have been an outbreak among the large numbers of refugees fleeing that country. Nevertheless, more than 1 million American lives have been lost despite our limited attempts at quarantine, while the Chinese economy was devastated by draconian efforts that were ultimately abandoned.

Sanitation can be learned but is difficult when armies are confined to close spaces and difficult terrain. Insect vectors can be attacked but are rarely eliminated. *Aedes* mosquitoes were controlled in Cuba during the Spanish-American War, but they continue to spread dengue fever. *Anopheles* mosquitoes are more adaptable, have a wider range, and remain difficult to control, a problem complicated by the toxicity of usual insecticides. Flies, fleas, lice, and ticks are ubiquitous and continue to spread disease. Climate change has expanded the range of disease-bearing insect vectors. Despite large-scale propaganda efforts and widespread spraying, insect-borne disease will almost certainly be a problem whenever troops are deployed in the tropics.

Drugs take time to develop, and microorganisms have a distressing ability to evolve around them. We face an expanding array of bacteria resistant to our best antibiotics, and effective antiviral drugs have proven elusive. Nonetheless, drugs are an advantage when one side has them and the other does not, so pharmacology and drug production will be key in future wars.

Vaccines can also provide an asymmetric advantage. They have the greatest impact when one side is immune and the other is not. A country with a vigorous, productive biomedical research community and an effective public health service will have a significant strategic advantage.

As recently as the mid-1970s infectious diseases were seen, even by the most respected academicians, as largely conquered.[4] A century of successful sanitary engineering, vaccines, and antibiotics had done their job. A series of epidemics and pandemics beginning with HIV/AIDS in 1981 and continuing through new strains of influenza, the novel coronaviruses SARS and MERS, drug-resistant tuberculosis, Zika, and COVID-19 have disabused us of that misconception. As much as we would like to believe that we have the tools to control the microorganisms that share our space, they greatly outnumber us and are disturbingly clever at outwitting us. Infectious disease will remain a major element of both public health and military strategy.

NOTES

INTRODUCTION

1. Hans Zinsser, *Rats, Lice, and History: Being a Study in Biography, Which, after Twelve Preliminary Chapters Indispensable for the Preparation of the Lay Reader, Deals with the Life History of Typhus Fever* (Boston: Little, Brown and Company, 1934), 132.

CHAPTER 1. IMMUNOLOGY

1. Stanhope Bayne-Jones, *The Evolution of Preventive Medicine in the United States Army, 1607–1939* (Washington, D.C.: Office of the Surgeon General, Department of the Army, 1968), 55.
2. *Variola minor*, described in Jamaica in 1863, is a considerably less lethal disease, with a mortality rate of approximately 1 percent, but as far as we know it did not exist in the North American colonies in the eighteenth century.
3. John Duffy, *Epidemics in Colonial America* (Baton Rouge: Louisiana State University Press, 1953), 20.
4. Duffy, *Epidemics in Colonial America*, 36.
5. Duffy, *Epidemics in Colonial America*, 104.
6. The procedure was initially too expensive for all but the wealthy.
7. The letter is currently held by the British Museum.
8. Otho Beall and Richard Shryock, *Cotton Mather: First Significant Figure in American Medicine* (Baltimore: Johns Hopkins University Press, 1954), 88.
9. Tony Williams, *The Pox and the Covenant: Mather, Franklin, and the Epidemic That Changed America's Destiny* (Naperville, IL: Sourcebooks, 2010), 69.
10. Duffy, *Epidemics in Colonial America*, 29.
11. Benjamin Franklin changed his mind in 1736 after his four-year-old son Francis died of smallpox. To the end of his life, he regretted not having inoculated the boy. He later published an editorial in the *Pennsylvania Gazette* citing Boston's 3 percent mortality from inoculation versus 25 percent from natural disease, although it must be remembered that the 25 percent is from people who actually had the disease and a truer comparison would be to the

entire susceptible population. He also published in the *Gazette* debunking the rumor that his son had died from inoculation. By the time of the Revolution Franklin was an ardent advocate for inoculation.

12. John Blake, "Smallpox Inoculation in Colonial Boston," *Journal of the History of Medicine and the Allied Sciences* 8 (1953): 283–300.

13. Blake, "Smallpox Inoculation in Colonial Boston," 297.

14. Blake, "Smallpox Inoculation in Colonial Boston," 297.

15. David Van Zwanenberg, "The Suttons and the Business of Inoculation," *Medical History* 22 (1978): 71–82

16. Elizabeth Fenn, *Pox Americana: The Great Smallpox Epidemic of 1775–1782* (New York: Hill and Wang, 2001), 39.

17. "Bill Concerning Inoculation for Smallpox, 27 December 1777," accessed January 2, 2021, https://founders.archives.gov/documents/Jefferson/01-02-02 -0040.

18. Lee fully expected to command the Continental Army but accepted being second in command at Boston when Massachusetts Maj. Gen. Artemas Ward resigned. He went on to command the successful repulse of the British invasion of Charleston before being captured by Banastre Tarleton. He was freed in a prisoner exchange in 1778. He was frequently critical of Washington's ability to command and was suspended from the army by a court-martial after a failed assault during the Battle of Monmouth. He left the military and died of a fever in Philadelphia in 1782.

19. Schuyler (1733–1804) had planned the Quebec invasion but was too sick to accompany the troops. He commanded the Northern Army until being replaced by Gen. Horatio Gates before the Battle of Saratoga. After the Revolution, he served as senator from New York. Of his fifteen children, one daughter, Angelica, was courted by Alexander Hamilton and another, Eliza, married him.

20. Washington's acceptance speech to Congress, Washington, D.C., 1921–26, Vol. II, 92. Quoted by *Continental Congress Journals, 1774–1789.*

21. Robert Middlekauff, *The Glorious Cause: The American Revolution, 1763–1789* (New York: Oxford University Press, 1982), 293.

22. James Thomas Flexner, *George Washington in the American Revolution (1775–1783)* (Boston: Little, Brown and Company, 1967), 37.

23. Middlekauff, *Glorious Cause*, 301.

24. Ann M. Becker, "Smallpox at the Siege of Boston: 'Vigilance against This Most Dangerous Enemy,'" *Historical Journal of Massachusetts* 45 (2017): 43–75.

25. "Washington in Barbados," accessed November 30, 2020, founders.archives .gov/Washington/01-01-02-0002-0004.

26. Becker, "Smallpox at the Siege of Boston," 51.

27. "From George Washington to John Hancock, 4 December 1775," accessed November 22, 2020, https://founders.archives.gov/documents/Washington /03-02-02-0437.

28. Catalog.archives.gov/id/824626. Record group 360. Accessed November 20, 2020.

29. "Washington to Hancock , 11 December 1775," accessed November 20, 2020, https://founders.archives.gov/?q=Washington%20to%20%20Hancock%20 Author%3A%22Washington%2C%20George%22&s=1111311113&r=91.

30. "Washington to Reed, 15 December 1775," accessed November 20, 2020, https://founders.archives.gov/?q=%20Period%3A%22Revolutionary%20 War%22%20Dates-From%3A1775-12-14%20Dates-To%3A1775-12 -18&s=1111311111&r=11.

31. Suspicion that the British were using smallpox as a bioweapon was not confined to Boston. Americans in Quebec were convinced that Sir Guy Carleton had done the same. Josiah Bartlet thought Tories in New Hampshire had as well.

32. "General Orders, 13 March 1776," accessed November 24, 2020, https:// founders.archives.gov/documents/Washington/03-03-02-0336.

33. Oscar Reiss, *Medicine and the American Revolution* (Jefferson, NC: McFarland, 1998), 88.

34. Fenn, *Pox Americana*, 88.

35. New York was allotted one major general and one brigadier. Montgomery doubted Schuyler had enough experience for the senior post but agreed to take the second spot when the New York Provisional Congress disagreed. When he passed through New York in June, Washington confirmed Schuyler as commander of the Northern Army with Montgomery as his second in command.

36. Reiss, *Medicine and the American Revolution*, 91.

37. Isaac Senter, *The Journal of Isaac Senter, Physician and Surgeon to the Troops Detached from the American Army Encamped at Cambridge, Mass. On a Secret Expedition against Quebec under the Command of Col. Benedict Arnold in September 1775* (Philadelphia: Historical Society of Pennsylvania, 1846), 21.

38. Senter, *Journal of Isaac Senter*, 22.

39. Senter, *Journal of Isaac Senter*, 28.

40. Fenn, *Pox Americana*, 64.

41. J. J. Henry, *Arnold's Campaign against Canada* (Albany, NY: Joel Munsell, 1877), 2–3.

42. Mary Gillett, *The Army Medical Department: 1775–1818* (Washington, D.C.: Center of Military History, United States Army, 1981), 59.

43. Gillett, *Army Medical Department*, 60.

44. Richard Blanco, "Military Medicine in Northern New York, 1776–1777," *New York History* 63 (1982): 39–58.

45. Francis R. Packard, *History of Medicine in the United States*, vol. 1 (New York: Paul B. Hoeber, 1931), 549.
46. John Lacey, "Memoirs," *Pennsylvania Magazine of Historical Biography* 25 (1901): 203–204.
47. Fenn, *Pox Americana*, 69.
48. "Daniel Kimball's Revolutionary War Journal of the March to Quebec," accessed November 20, 2020, https://catalog.archives.gov/id/23914415.
49. Rebecca Seaman, ed., *Epidemics and War: The Impact of Disease on Major Conflicts in History* (Santa Barbara, CA: ABC-CLIO, 2018), 151.
50. Fenn, *Pox Americana*, 131.
51. John Hancock offered his home to Martha Washington as well as his household staff to care for her. She declined and took up residence with the cabinet maker Benjamin Randolph in quarters vacated by Thomas Jefferson.
52. Packard, *History of Medicine in the United States*, 83.
53. "To George Washington from William Shippen Jr., 25 January 1777," accessed December 28, 2020, https://founders.archives.gov/documents/Washington/03-08-02-0163.
54. "From George Washington to Major General Horatio Gates, 5–6 February 1777," accessed December 27, 2020, https://founders.archives.gov/documents/Washington/03-08-02-0267.
55. "Washington to William Shippen Jr., 6 February 1777," accessed December 27, 2020, https://founders.archives.gov/documents/Washington/03-08-02-0281.
56. "Washington to William Shippen, 6 February 1777."
57. Washington to Congress from Morristown; Packard, *History of Medicine*, 578.
58. From the *Journals of the Continental Congress* cited in William O. Owen, *The Medical Department of the United States Army during the Period of the Revolution (1776–1786)* (New York: Paul B. Hoeber, 1920), 57.
59. Fenn, *Pox Americana*, 95.
60. Owen, *Medical Department of the United States Army*, 98.
61. Gillett, *Army Medical Department*, 125.

CHAPTER 2. ECOLOGY

1. Richard Shryock, "A Medical Perspective on the Civil War," *American Quarterly* 14 (1962): 161–73.
2. An exception was in Major General William Tecumseh Sherman's campaign in Georgia and South Carolina. His men may have remained healthy because they were constantly on the move.
3. James Longstreet, *From Manassas to Appomattox: Memoirs of the Civil War in America* (Secaucus, NJ: Blue and Grey Press, 1984), 64–162.

4. George Worthington Adams, *Doctors in Blue: The Medical History of the Union Army in the Civil War* (Baton Rouge: Louisiana State University Press, 1952), 13.

5. P. M. Ashburn, *A History of the Medical Department of the United States Army* (Boston: Houghton Mifflin Company, 1929), 87.

6. Adams, *Doctors in Blue*, 8.

7. Adams, *Doctors in Blue*, 21.

8. "Medical Bureau of the Army," *New York Times*, November 25, 1861, 4.

9. Mary Gillett, *The Army Medical Department: 1818–1865* (Washington, D.C.: Center of Military History, United States Army, 1987), 179.

10. Alfred Jay Bollet, *Civil War Medicine: Challenges and Triumphs* (Tucson, AZ: Galen Press, 2002), 18.

11. William A. Hammond, "Annual Report of the Surgeon General, U.S.A.," *Boston Medical and Surgical Journal* 67 (1863): 437–43.

12. Ashburn, *History of the Medical Department*, 88.

13. Robert Denny, *Civil War Medicine: Care and Comfort of the Wounded* (New York: Sterling Publishing, 1995), 84.

14. Adams, *Doctors in Blue*, 159.

15. J. J. Woodward, "Typho-Malarial Fever: Is It a Special Type of Fever? Remarks Introductory to the Discussion of the Question, Section of Medicine, International Medical Congress, Philadelphia 1876," reprint, accessed November 9, 2021, https://collections.nlm.nih.gov/catalog/nlm:nlmuid-9609653-bk.

16. Joseph Janvier Woodward, *Outlines of the Chief Camp Diseases of the United States Armies as Observed during the Present War* (Philadelphia: Lippincott, 1863; reprinted San Francisco: Norman Publishing, 1992), 28.

17. H. H. Cunningham, *Doctors in Gray: The Confederate Medical Service* (Baton Rouge: Louisiana State University Press, 1958), 186.

18. Bollet, *Civil War Medicine*, 240.

19. Cunningham, *Doctors in Gray*, 17.

20. "Medicine as a Determining Factor in War," *Scientific Monthly* 9 (July 1919): 93, https://www.jstor.org/stable/6472.

21. "Medicine as a Determining Factor in War," 91, 93.

22. Cited in "Woodward's Report to the Surgeon General U.S. Army," *Confederate States Medical and Surgical Journal* 1 (January 1864).

23. Paul Steiner, *Disease in the Civil War: National Biological Warfare in 1861–1865* (Springfield, IL: Charles C. Thomas, 1968), 4.

24. Joseph Barnes, *Medical and Surgical History of the War of the Rebellion*, Medical Volume, Part 1 (Washington, D.C.: Government Printing Office, 1870), 636.

25. Bollet, *Civil War Medicine*, 262.

26. Bollet, *Civil War Medicine*, 269.

27. Cunningham, *Doctors in Gray*, 188.

28. Cunningham, *Doctors in Gray*, 190.

29. Frank Freemon, *Gangrene and Glory: Medical Care during the American Civil War* (Urbana: University of Illinois Press, 2001), 210.

30. Denny, *Civil War Medicine*, 63.

31. Jeffrey S. Sartin, "Infectious Diseases during the Civil War: The Triumph of the 'Third Army,'" *Clinical Infectious Diseases* 16 (April 1993): 580–84.

32. *Confederate States Medical and Surgical Journal* 1, no. 6 (July 1864).

33. Cunningham, *Doctors in Gray*, 261.

34. Stanhope Bayne-Jones, *The Evolution of Preventive Medicine in the United States Army, 1607–1939* (Washington, D.C.: Office of the Surgeon General, Department of the Army, 1968), 200.

35. Bollet, *Civil War Medicine*, 295.

36. See H. Leon Greene, *The Confederate Yellow Fever Conspiracy: The Germ Warfare Plot of Luke Pryor Blackburn, 1864–1865* (Jefferson, NC: McFarland, 2019), for a full description of the episode.

37. Barnes, *Medical and Surgical History*, 636.

38. Bayne-Jones, *Evolution of Preventive Medicine*, 99.

39. Charles Smart, *Medical and Surgical History of the War of the Rebellion, Medical Volume, Third Part* (Washington, D.C.: Government Printing Office, 1888), 11.

40. *Confederate States Journal* 1, no. 9 (1864).

41. Frank Hastings Hamilton, *A Practical Treatise on Military Surgery* (New York: Balliere Brothers, 1861; reprinted by Norman Publishing, 1989), 201.

42. Woodward, *Outlines*, 36.

43. Woodward, *Outlines*, 167.

44. Woodward, *Outlines*, 162.

45. Barnes, *Medical and Surgical History*, 636.

46. Stewart Brooks, *Civil War Medicine* (Springfield, IL: Charles C. Thomas, 1966), 119.

47. "Grand Summary of the Sick and Wounded of the Confederate States Army during the Years 1861 and 1862," *Confederate States Journal* 1 (1864): 139–40.

48. Woodward, *Outlines*, 168.

49. Cunningham, *Doctors in Gray*, 192.

50. Jenish Bhandari, Pawan Theda, and Elizabeth DeVos, "Typhoid Fever," accessed February 23, 2021, www.ncbi.nlm.nih.gov/books/NBK557513/.

51. Woodward, *Outlines*, 50.

52. Woodward, *Outlines*, 54.

53. Hamilton, *Practical Treatise on Military Surgery*, 201.

54. Bollet, *Civil War Medicine*, 273.

55. "Grand Summary of the Sick and Wounded," 139–40.

56. Adams, *Doctors in Blue*, 15.

57. Charles Stuart Tripler and George Curtis Blackman, *Hand-book for the Military Surgeon* (Cincinnati, OH: R. Clarke, 1861; reprinted by Norman Publishing, 1989), 10.

58. Tripler and Blackman, *Hand-book for the Military Surgeon*, 32.

59. For a full description of McClellan's typhoid and its result, see Ethan Rafuse, "Typhoid and Tumult: Lincoln's Response to General McClellan's Bout with Typhoid Fever," *Journal of the Abraham Lincoln Association* 18, no. 2 (1997): 1–16.

60. Steiner, *Disease in the Civil War*, 133.

61. Steiner, *Disease in the Civil War*, 139.

62. Shelby Foote, *The Civil War, a Narrative: Fort Sumter to Perryville* (New York: Random House, 1958), 493.

63. Gillett, *Army Medical Department*, 268.

64. Smart, *Medical and Surgical History*, 33.

65. Greene, *Confederate Yellow Fever Conspiracy*, 45.

66. Greene, *Confederate Yellow Fever Conspiracy*, 45. Note that these numbers are slightly greater than those given in the *Medical and Surgical History*.

67. "Medicine, a Determining Factor in War," *Science* 50 (July 1919): 8–11.

68. "Grand Summary of the Sick and Wounded," 139–40.

69. Greene, *Confederate Yellow Fever Conspiracy*, 45.

70. "Medicine, a Determining Factor in War," 8–11.

71. Abram Benenson, "Immunization and Military Medicine," *Reviews of Infectious Disease* 6 (January–February 1984): 1–12.

72. Assistant Surgeon J. J. Erwin of the 10th Ohio Volunteer Infantry quoted in Vincent J. Cirillo, *Bullets and Bacilli: The Spanish-American War and Military Medicine* (New Brunswick, NJ: Rutgers University Press, 1999), 68.

73. "The Typhoid Outbreak in the United States Military Camps during the Spanish War," *British Medical Journal* 2 (July 1905): 137–40.

74. Benenson, "Immunization and Military Medicine."

75. "Awful Suffering at Camp Thomas," *New York Times*, August 10, 1898.

76. Alexander Becker, "Typhoid Fever: Its Causes and Sources as Explained by the Germ Theory of Disease," reprinted from *The Boston Medical and Surgical Journal*, 1879, accessed November 15, 2021, https://collections.nlm.nih.gov/bookviewer?PID=nlm:nlmuid-101683349-bk.

77. Augusto Caillé, "Our Present Knowledge Concerning the Aetiology of Typhoid Fever," *New York Medical Journal*, January 19, 1889, reprint, accessed November 17, 2021, https://collections.nlm.nih.gov/catalog/nlm:nlmuid-101723401-bk.

78. Vincent J. Cirillo, *Bullets and Bacilli: The Spanish-American War and Military Medicine* (New Brunswick, NJ: Rutgers University Press, 1999), 66. Widal claimed 100 percent sensitivity and specificity.

79. Vincent Cirillo, "'The Patriotic Order': Sanitation and Typhoid Fever in the National Encampments during the Spanish-American War," *Army History* 49 (2000): 17–23.

80. P. M. Ashburn, *The Elements of Military Hygiene Especially Arranged for Officers and Men of the Line* (Boston: Houghton Mifflin Company, 1909), 51.

CHAPTER 3. A DIFFERENT APPROACH TO ECOLOGY

1. There is a sylvatic form of yellow fever that is endemic in forest monkeys and is carried by *Aedes* africanus and *Aedes* bromeliad. Those mosquitoes breed in cavities in the upper forest canopy and can infect humans venturing into the trees, typically in lumber harvesting. That has proven to be a very difficult source of yellow fever to control and accounts for its persistence in Africa and Amazonian South America and the fact that there are still about 200,000 cases of yellow fever in the world each year with about 30,000 deaths.

2. Thomas P. Monath, "Yellow Fever: An Update," *Lancet Infectious Diseases* 1 (2001): 11–20.

3. J. R. McNeill, "Yellow Jack and Geopolitics: Environment, Epidemics, and the Struggles for Empire in the American Tropics, 1640–1830," *Review (Fernand Braudel Center No. 4), The Environment and World History* 4 (2004): 343–64.

4. McNeill, "Yellow Jack and Geopolitics," has a full discussion of these events.

5. James Carroll, "Remarks on the History, Cause, and Mode of Transmission of Yellow Fever and the Occurrence of Similar Types of Fatal Fevers in Places Where Yellow Fever Is Not Known to Have Existed." Reprinted from *Journal of the Association of Military Surgeons of the United States* (Carlisle, PA: Association of Military Surgeons, 1903).

6. D. LaRoche, *Yellow Fever, Considered in Its Historical, Pathological, Etiological, and Therapeutic Relations*, vol. 2 (Philadelphia: Blanchard and Lea, 1855), 732.

7. Alvah H. Doty, "The Scientific Prevention of Yellow Fever," *North American Review* 167 (1898): 681–89.

8. Ironically, Nott was the physician who delivered William Gorgas.

9. Jari Vainio and Felicity Cutts, "Yellow Fever," from *World Health Organization. Division of Emerging and Other Communicable Diseases Surveillance and Control* (Geneva, 1998).

10. Howard A. Kelly, *Walter Reed and Yellow Fever* (Baltimore: Medical Standard Book Company, 1906), 64.

11. The applicant who finished first in that group was William Hammond, one of Miller's predecessors as surgeon general of the Army.

12. Finlay was christened Juan Carlos but subsequently reversed the order to Carlos Juan and was generally known by the first name only.

13. Cited in J. L. Sanchez, *Carlos Finlay: His Life and Work* (Havana, Cuba: Editorial José Marti, 1999), 190.

14. Martha Sternberg, *George Miller Sternberg: A Biography* (Chicago: American Medical Association, 1920), 109.

15. Sternberg, *George Miller Sternberg*, 279.

16. Albert Truby, *Memoir of Walter Reed: The Yellow Fever Episode* (New York: Paul B. Hoeber, 1943), 9.

17. Truby, *Memoir of Walter Reed*, 44.

18. Transcript of Philip Showalter Hench's interview of Jefferson Randolph Kean, June 5, 1946, Bos-folder 64:9, Philip S. Hench Walter Reed Yellow Fever Collection 1806–1995, Historical Collections, Claude Moore Health Sciences Library, University of Virginia.

19. William Osler, "Discussion of G. M. Sternberg, 'The Bacillus Icteroides (Sanarelli) and Bacillus x (Sternberg),'" *Transactions of the Association of American Physicians* 13 (1898): 71.

20. William Osler, *The Principles and Practice of Medicine* (New York: D. Appleton and Company, 1899), 183.

21. Margaret Warner, "Hunting the Yellow Fever Germ: The Principle and Practice of Etiological Proof in the Late Nineteenth Century," *Bulletin of the History of Medicine* 59 (1985): 361–82.

22. "Obituary, Surgeon General Walter Wyman," *Military Surgeon* 29 (December 1911): 699.

23. The quotations are cited in Mariola Espinosa, "The Threat from Havana: Southern Public Health, Yellow Fever, and the U.S. Intervention in the Cuban Struggle for Independence, 1878–1898," *Journal of Southern History* 72 (2006): 541–68.

24. Cited in Espinosa, "Threat from Havana."

25. Subsequent investigation, most notably by Admiral Hyman Rickover in 1974, concluded that the explosion was most likely caused by spontaneous combustion in a coal bunker and ignition of volatile firedamp gases.

26. Wood was contemporary with several other important figures in the yellow fever episode. He was commissioned in 1886, Kean in 1884, Gorgas in 1880, and Reed in 1875.

27. Jack McCallum, *Leonard Wood: Rough Rider, Surgeon, Architect of American Imperialism* (New York: New York University Press, 2006), 66.

28. Walter Reed asked to be assigned to Captain William Sampson's squadron, but Sternberg, no doubt unwilling to have his best researcher away from the laboratory, turned him down. His son Lawrence did, however, enlist and made the military a career. He was eventually commissioned and retired a major general.

29. Osler, *Principles and Practice*, 182.

30. Kelly, *Walter Reed and Yellow Fever*, 95.

31. Enrique Chaves-Carballo, "Carlos Finlay and Yellow Fever: Triumph over Adversity," *Military Medicine* 10 (2005): 881–85.

32. "The Prevention of Yellow Fever," *British Medical Journal* 2 (1901): 1104.

33. Memorandum from Surgeon General to Adjutant General, May 13, 1900. NARA Record Group 112. Italics added.

34. Aristedes Agramonte, "The Inside History of a Great Medical Discovery," *Scientific Monthly* 1 (1915): 209–37.

35. Transcript of Philip Showalter Hench's interview with Jefferson Randolph Kean, January 6, 1944, Box-folder 64:2; transcript of Philip Showalter Hench's interview with Jefferson Randolph Kean.

36. Agramonte, "Inside History of a Great Medical Discovery."

37. Agramonte, "Inside History of a Great Medical Discovery."

38. In an ironic coincidence, Reed's son Lawrence had been on the jury that sent Arthur Hoskins to jail.

39. Statement by Aristides Agramonte concerning work of the U.S. Yellow Fever Commission, August 31, 1908, Box-folder 29:61, Philip S. Hench Walter Reed Yellow Fever Collection 1806–1995, Historical Collections, Claude Moore Health Sciences Library, University of Virginia.

40. John Pierce and Jim Writer, *Yellow Jack: How Yellow Fever Ravaged America and Walter Reed Discovered Its Deadly Secrets* (Hoboken, NJ: Wiley, 2005), 145.

41. He was also said to have been ordered back by Sternberg to complete the report of the Typhoid Commission on which he had served with Victor Vaughan and Edward Shakespeare, but no such order has ever been found.

42. Lawrence Altman, *Who Goes First: The Story of Self-Experimentation in Medicine* (New York: Random House, 1986), 148.

43. Altman, *Who Goes First*, 148.

44. Cushing Harvey, *The Life of Sir William Osler*, vol. 1 (Oxford: Clarendon Press, 1926), 523.

45. Truby, *Memoir of Walter Reed*, 104.

46. Agramonte, "Inside History of a Great Medical Discovery."

47. McCallum, *Leonard Wood*, 170–71.

48. William Bean, *Walter Reed: A Biography* (Charlottesville: University Press of Virginia, 1982), 147.

49. Both Folk and Jernegan volunteered for later experiments, and both contracted yellow fever proving they were not immune at the time of the "infected clothing" experiment.

50. Moran's Story, circa 1937. Box-folder 34:22, Philip S. Hench Walter Reed Yellow Fever Collection 1806–1995, Historical Collections, Claude Moore Health Sciences Library, University of Virginia.

51. Akhil Mehra, "Politics of Participation: Walter Reed's Yellow Fever Experiments," *American Medical Association Journal of Ethics* 11 (2009): 326–30.

52. Agramonte, "Inside History of a Great Medical Discovery."

53. Bean, *Walter Reed*, 153.

54. Building No. 2 was destroyed in a storm. The other building survived as a ruin.

55. Moran's Story, Hench papers.

56. John Moran, "Mosquitoes and Yellow Fever," *British Medical Journal* 1 (1901): 1102.

57. George Sternberg, "The Transmission of Yellow Fever by Mosquitoes," *Popular Science Monthly*, July 1901, cited in Truby, *Memoir of Walter Reed*, 90.

58. Kean to Reed, October 13, 1901, Philip S. Hench Walter Reed Yellow Fever Collection 1806–1995, Historical Collections, Claude Moore Health Sciences Library, University of Virginia.

59. John H. Andrus, "An Episode from *Big Moments in a Little Life*, circa 1940–1955," Box-folder 65:10, Philip S. Hench Walter Reed Yellow Fever Collection 1806–1995, Historical Collections, Claude Moore Health Sciences Library, University of Virginia.

60. Andrus, "Episode from *Big Moments in a Little Life*."

61. From Chief Surgeons Office Headquarters Department of Western Cuba, Quemados, October 13, 1900, Philip S. Hench Walter Reed Yellow Fever Collection 1806–1995, Historical Collections, Claude Moore Health Sciences Library, University of Virginia.

62. Letter from Jefferson Randolph Kean to Philip Showalter Hench, February 5, 1947, Box-folder 64:13, Philip S. Hench Walter Reed Yellow Fever Collection 1806–1995, Historical Collections, Claude Moore Health Sciences Library, University of Virginia.

63. "Experimental Yellow Fever," *American Medicine*, July 6, 1901, and "The Etiology of Yellow Fever—A Supplemental Note, *American Medicine*, February 22, 1902.

CHAPTER 4. QUARANTINE

1. Michael Worobey, Guan-Zhu Han, and Andrew Rambaut, "Genesis and Pathogenesis of the 1918 Pandemic H1N1 Influenza Virus," *Proceedings of the National Academy of Sciences of the United States of America* 22 (June 2014): 8107–112.

2. Bruno Lina, "History of Pandemics," in *Paleomicrobioilogy*, D. Raoult and M. Drancourt, eds. (Berlin: Springer-Verlag, 2008), 199–211.

3. Michelle Rozo and Gigi Kwik Gronvall, "The Reemergent 1977 H1 N1 Strain and the Gain-of-Function Debate," *mBio*, accessed May 3, 2021, https://journals.asm.org/doi/10.1128/mBio.01013-15.

4. Jeffery K. Taubenberger and David M. Morens, "1918 Influenza: The Mother of All Pandemics," *Emerging Infectious Diseases* 12 (2006): 15–22.

5. His residents coined a poem:

    > *Nobody knows where Popsy eats*
    > *Nobody knows where Popsy sleeps*
    > *Nobody knows who Popsy keeps*
    > *But Popsy*

6. M. W. Ireland, *Report of the Surgeon General U.S. Army to the Secretary of War, 1919* (Washington, D.C.: Government Printing Office, 1919), 38.

7. John Barry, *The Great Influenza: The Epic Story of the Deadliest Plague in History* (New York: Penguin Books, 2004), 310.

8. Carol Byerly, *Fever of War: The Influenza Epidemic in the U.S. Army during World War I* (New York: New York University Press, 2005), 45.

9. Dorothy Ann Petit and Janice Bailie, *A Cruel Wind: American Experiences in the Pandemic Influenza; 1918–1920, A Social History* (Murfreesboro, TN: Timberlane Books, 2008), 175.

10. Kansas Historical Society, "Camp Funston," accessed April 13, 2021, http://KSHS.org/kansaspedia/camp_funston/166.92.

11. Laura Spinney, *Pale Rider: The Spanish Influenza of 1918 and How It Changed the World* (New York: Public Affairs, 1917), 37.

12. Merrit Ireland, *Medical Department of the United States Army in the World War*, vol. 9, *Communicable Diseases* (Washington, D.C.: U.S. Army, 1929), 159.

13. Taubenberger and Morens, "1918 Influenza."

14. Alfred Crosby, *Epidemic and Peace* (Westport, CT: Greenwood Press, 1976), 25.

15. J. S. Oxford, "World War I May Have Allowed the Emergence of 'Spanish' Influenza," *Lancet: Infectious Diseases* 2, no. 2 (2002): 111–14.

16. Mark Osborne Humphries, "Paths of Infection: The First World War and the Origins of the 1918 Influenza Pandemic," *War in History* 1 (2014): 55–81; and

Christopher Langford, "Did the 1918–19 Influenza Pandemic Originate in China?," *Population and Development Review* 31 (2005): 473–505.

17. Royal College of Physicians, "Prevention and Treatment of Influenza," *British Medical Journal* 2 (November 16, 1918): 546.

18. P. M. Ashburn, *A History of the Medical Department of the United States Army* (Boston: Houghton Mifflin Company, 1929), 317.

19. The numbers continued to balloon: 297,000 in June, more than 300,000 in July, and 286,000 in August.

20. Influenza Committee of the Advisory Board, "A Report on the Influenza Epidemic in the British Armies in France, 1918," *British Medical Journal* 2 (November 9, 1918): 505–509.

21. Barry, *Great Influenza*, 174.

22. Gina Kolata, *Influenza: The Story of the Great Influenza Pandemic of 1918 and the Search for the Virus That Caused It* (New York: Farrar, Straus and Giroux, 1999), 11.

23. Barry, *Great Influenza*, 170.

24. Andrew T. Price-Smith, *Contagion and Chaos: Disease, Ecology, and National Security in the Era of Globalization* (Cambridge, MA: MIT Press, 2009), 68.

25. Harvey Cushing, *From a Surgeon's Journal* (Boston: Little, Brown, and Company, 1937), 396.

26. Cushing, *Journal*, 411.

27. Erich von Ludendorff, *Ludendorff's Own Story*, vol. 2 (New York: Harper and Bros., 1919), 277.

28. See David Zabecki, *The German 1918 Offensives: A Case Study in the Operational Level of War* (London: Routledge, 2006).

29. Kolata, *Influenza*, 81.

30. G. D. Shanks, G. J. Milinovich, M. Waller, and A. C. A. Clements, "Spatio-Temporal Investigation of the 1918 Influenza Pandemic in Military Populations Indicates Two Different Viruses," *Epidemiology and Infection* 143 (July 2015): 1816–25.

31. Humphries, "Paths of Infection."

32. *Public Health Reports (1876–1970)*, September 6, 1918, 1530.

33. Crosby, *Epidemic and Peace*, 38.

34. Crosby, *Epidemic and Peace*, 38.

35. Carol Byerly, "The U.S. Military and the Influenza Pandemic of 1918–19, *Public Health Reports (Washington, D.C.: 1974)* 125 (April 2010); *Supplement 3: The 1918–1919 Influenza Pandemic in the United States* (April 2010): 82–91.

36. Nick McGrath, "Fort Devens Massachusetts," *On Point* 20 (2015): 44–47.

37. Victor C. Vaughan, *Doctor's Memories* (Indianapolis, IN: Bobbs-Merrill Company, 1926), 383–84.

38. Vaughan, *Doctor's Memories*, 431–32.
39. Kolata, *Influenza*, 17.
40. Barry, *Great Influenza*, 189.
41. Edgar Sydenstricker, "Variations in Case Fatality during the Influenza Epidemic of 1918," *Public Health Reports (1896–1970)* 36 (September 9, 1921): 2201–10.
42. Ashburn, *History of the Medical Department*, 320.
43. "War Department Special Regulation No. 28," *Sanitary Regulations and Control of Communicable Diseases* (Washington, D.C.: Government Printing Office, 1917), 7.
44. Crosby, *Epidemic and Peace*, 31.
45. Byerly, "U.S. Military and the Influenza."
46. Byerly, "U.S. Military and the Influenza," 752.
47. Byerly, "U.S. Military and the Influenza," 768.
48. Kathleen Fargey, "The Deadliest Enemy," *Army History* 111 (Spring 2019): 24–39.
49. Memorandum No. 449, September 30, 1918 from Headquarters, Camp Humphreys. Cited in L. Col. H. W. Brenner, "Report of Epidemic 'Spanish Influenza' Which Occurred at Camp A. A. Humphreys, VA during September and October, 1918." RG 112 Records of the Office of the Surgeon General National Archives, accessed April 15, 2021, https://www.influenzaarchive.org.
50. David Morens and Jeffery Taubenberger, "Predominant Role of Bacterial Pneumonia as a Cause of Death in Pandemic Influenza: Implications for Pandemic Influenza Preparedness," *Journal of Infectious Disease* 198 (2008): 962–70.
51. Petit and Bailie, *Cruel Wind*, 371.
52. N. R. Grist, "Pandemic Influenza," *British Medical Journal* 2 (December 1979): 1632.
53. Stuart McGuire, *History of U.S. Army Base Hospital No. 45 in the Great War* (Richmond, VA: William Byrd Press, 1924), 252.
54. Harold Barclay, *A Doctor in France, 1917–1919* (New York: Privately printed, 1923), 130.
55. Grist, "Pandemic Influenza," 1632.
56. Lyn McDonald, *The Roses of No Man's Land* (New York: Atheneum, 1980), 289.
57. Crosby, *Epidemic and Peace*, 124.
58. George Soper, "The Influenza Pandemic in the American Army Camps during September and October 1918," *Science, New Series* 48 (November 8, 1918): 451–56.
59. Soper, "Influenza Pandemic," 64.
60. McDonald, *Roses of No Man's Land*, 292.

61. Edgar Faulkner, "Disappearing Doughboys: The American Expeditionary Force's Straggler Crisis in the Meuse-Argonne," *Army History* (Spring 2012): 7–25.

62. Byerly, *Fever of War*, 55.

63. I. L. Lumsden, "Influenza: Avoid It and Prevent Its Spread," *Public Health Reports (1896–1970)* 33 (October 1918): 731–32.

64. Stephen Morse, "Influenza: Studying the Lessons of History," *Proceedings of the National Academy of Sciences of the United States of America* 104 (May 2007): 7313–14.

65. John Eyler, "The Fog of Research: Influenza Vaccine Trials during the 1918–19 Pandemic," *Journal of the History of Medicine and the Allied Sciences* 64 (October 2009): 401–28.

66. W. B. Leishman, "Vaccines for Influenza," *British Medical Journal* 2 (October 26, 1918): 470.

67. Julian Navarro, "Influenza in 1918: An Epidemic in Images," *Public Health Reports Supplement 3* 125 (2010): 9–14.

68. Eyler, "Fog of Research."

69. Byerly, *Fever of War*, 49.

70. Kolata, *Influenza*, 58.

71. Eyler, "Fog of Research."

72. Jeffery Taubenberger, "Seeking the 1918 Spanish Influenza Virus," *American Society of Microbiology News* 65 (July 1999).

73. Barry, *Great Influenza*, 239.

74. *Report of the Surgeon General U.S. Army to the Secretary of War: 1919*, 43.

75. Fargey, "Deadliest Enemy."

76. Fargey, "Deadliest Enemy."

77. *Report of the Surgeon General U.S. Army to the Secretary of War: 1919*, 42.

78. Jose Sanchez, "Influenza in the U.S. Military: An Overview," *Journal of Infectious Diseases and Treatment* 2 (2016): 1–7.

79. Howard G. Coombs, "The Influenza Pandemic of 1918: Military Observations for Today," in *COVID-19: NATO in the Age of Pandemics*, Thierry Tardy, ed. (NATO Defense College), accessed April 8, 2021, https://www.jstor.org/stable/resrep25148.13#metadata_info_tab_contents.

80. Fargey, "Deadliest Enemy."

CHAPTER 5. PHARMACOLOGY

1. Arthur M. Smith and Craig Hooper, "The Mosquito Can Be More Dangerous Than the Mortar Round: The Obligations of Command," *Naval War College Review* 58 (Winter 2005): 77–87.

2. Smith and Hooper, "The Mosquito Can Be More Dangerous."
3. Richard Tregaskis, *Guadalcanal Diary* (New York: Random House), 1943.
4. J. A. Sinton, "Malaria in War," *Ulster Medical Journal* 15(1946): 3–28.
5. "World Malaria Report, 2021," World Health Organization, accessed April 13, 2022, https://www.who.int/teams/global-malaria-programme/reports/world -malaria-report-2021.
6. K. W. Kelvin and Kwok-Yung Yuen, "In Memory of Patrick Manson, Founding Father of Tropical Medicine and the Discovery of Vector-Borne Infections," *Emerging Microbes and Infections* (2012), accessed July 14, 2021, https://www .ncbi.nlm.nih.gov/pmc/articles/PMC3630944/.
7. Dennis Worthen, "The National Quinine Pool: When Quinine Went to War," *Pharmacy in History* 38 (1996): 143–47.
8. Willian Fletcher and K. Kanagarayer, "Plasmochin in the Treatment of Malaria," *Indian Medical Gazette* 62 (1927): 499–506.
9. N. H. Fairley, "Researches in Paludine (M.4888) in Malaria," *Transactions of the Royal Society of Tropical Medicine and Hygiene* 40 (October 1946): 105–51.
10. Peter Weina, "From Atabrine in World War II to Mefloquine in Somalia: The Role of Education in Preventive Medicine," *Military Medicine* 163 (September 1998): 635–39.
11. Howland Sargeant and Henrietta Creamer, "Enemy Patents," *Law and Contemporary Problems, Vol. 1: Enemy Property* 11 (1945): 92–108.
12. H. P. Willmott, *Empires in the Balance: Japanese and Allied Pacific Strategies to April 1942* (Annapolis: Naval Institute Press, 1982).
13. Ronald H. Spector, *Eagle against the Sun: The American War with Japan* (New York: Free Press, 1985).
14. James O. Gillespie, "Malaria and the Defense of Bataan," in *Preventive Medicine in World War II, Volume VI, Communicable Diseases, Malaria*, John Boyd Coates, ed. (Washington, D.C.: Office of the Surgeon General, Department of the Army, 1963), 507.
15. Willmott, *Empires in the Balance*, 386.
16. Spector, *Eagle against the Sun*, 115.
17. Gillespie, "Malaria and the Defense of Bataan," 511.
18. Gillespie, "Malaria and the Defense of Bataan," 503.
19. Gillespie, "Malaria and the Defense of Bataan," 510.
20. John W. H. Rehn, "China-Burma-India Theater," in *Preventive Medicine in World War II , Volume VI, Communicable Diseases, Malaria*, John Boyd Coates, ed. (Washington, D.C.: Office of the Surgeon General, Department of the Army, 1963), 356.
21. Rehn, "China-Burma-India Theater," 367.
22. Spector, *Eagle against the Sun*, 332.

23. Weina, "From Atabrine in World War II," 635–39.
24. Derek M. Salmi, "Slim's Burma Campaign," in *Slim Chance: The Pivotal Role of Air Mobility in the Burma Campaign* (April 1, 2014), Air University Press, accessed June 1, 2021, http://www.jstor.com/stable/resrep13911.9.
25. Rehn, "China-Burma-India Theater," 393.
26. Weina, "From Atabrine in World War II."
27. Robert J. T. Joy, "Malaria in American Troops in the South and Southwest Pacific in World War II," *Medical History* 43 (1999): 192–207.
28. Salmi, "Slim's Burma Campaign."
29. Wingate had died in a plane crash in March as well.
30. Christopher Kolakowski, "Courage, and Devotion to Duty," *Army History* 116 (Summer 2020): 6–23.
31. Rehn, "China-Burma-India Theater," 374.
32. Rehn, "China-Burma-India Theater," 395.
33. Maurice Matloff and Edwin M. Snell, *Strategic Planning for Coalition Warfare, 1942–1942* (Washington, D.C.: Office of the Chief of Military History, 1953), 162–64.
34. H. D. Steward, *Recollections of a Regimental Medical Officer* (Melbourne: Melbourne University Press, 1983), 22. It should be noted that mortality from malaria among Japanese troops in New Guinea has elsewhere been cited as less than 3 percent. George Dennis Shanks, "Decreased Mortality of *Falciparum* Malaria in Anemic Prisoners of War?," *American Journal of Tropical Medicine and Hygiene* 6 (December 2020): 2171–73.
35. Thomas Hart, "Southwest Pacific Area," in *Preventative Medicine in World War II, Volume VI, Communicable Diseases, Malaria*, John Boyd Coates, ed. (Washington, D.C.: Office of the Surgeon General, Department of the Army, 1963), 573.
36. John T. Greenwood, "The Fight against Malaria in the Papua and New Guinea Campaigns," *Army History* 59 (Summer–Fall 2003): 16–28.
37. Albert Cowdrey, *Fighting for Life: American Military Medicine in World War II* (New York: Free Press, 1994), 77.
38. Hart, "Southwest Pacific Area," 568.
39. Mary Ellen Condon-Rall, "Allied Cooperation in Malaria Prevention and Control: The World War II Southwest Pacific Experience," *Journal of the History of Medicine and Allied Sciences* 46 (October 1991): 493–513.
40. Cowdrey, *Fighting for Life*, 182.
41. Greenwood, "Fight against Malaria," 57.
42. Paul Russell, "Introduction," in *Preventive Medicine in World War II , Volume VI, Communicable Diseases, Malaria*, John Boyd Coates, ed. (Washington, D.C.: Office of the Surgeon General, Department of the Army, 1963), 2.

43. Greenwood, "Fight against Malaria."

44. Greenwood, "Fight against Malaria."

45. Seth Paltzer, "The Other Foe: The U.S. Army's Fight against Malaria in the Pacific Theater, 1942–1945," *Army History* (Winter 2016): 6–12.

46. Weina, "From Atabrine in World War II."

47. Weina, "From Atabrine in World War II."

48. Bernard Rostker, "Providing for Casualties of War," in *The American Experience in World War II* (Santa Monica, CA: RAND Corporation), accessed June 2, 2021, https://www.jstor.org/stable/10.7249/j.ctt2tt90p.

49. Oliver R. McCoy, "War Department Provisions for Malaria Control," in *Preventive Medicine in World War II, Volume VI, Communicable Diseases, Malaria*, John Boyd Coates, ed. (Washington, D.C.: Office of the Surgeon General, Department of the Army, 1963), 15.

50. McCoy, "War Department Provisions for Malaria Control," 18.

51. Fairley, "Researches in Paludrine (M.4888) in Malaria," 105–51.

52. All three sulfa drugs tried were ineffective.

53. Condon-Rall, "Allied Cooperation in Malaria Prevention."

54. Georgina Kenyon, "Australian Army Infected Troops and Internees in Second World War," *British Medical Journal* 318 (May 1999): 1233.

55. Hart, "Southwest Pacific Area," 562.

56. William L. Laurence, "New Drugs to Combat Malaria Are Tested in Prisons for Army," *New York Times*, March 5, 1945.

57. Nathaniel Comfort, "The Prisoner as Model Organism: Malaria Research at Stateville Penitentiary," *Studies in History, Philosophy, Biology, and Biomedical Science* 40 (September 2009): 190–203.

58. Bernard E. Harcourt, "Making Willing Bodies: The University of Chicago Human Experiments at Stateville Penitentiary," *Social Research* 78 (Summer 2011): 443–78.

59. Harcourt, "Making Willing Bodies."

60. Before penicillin was widely available to treat syphilis, *Vivax* malaria was used to induce high fevers, which had been shown to lessen symptoms and slow progression of the venereal disease.

61. He claimed to have helped write eighteen of the twenty-two published papers from the Stateville experiments.

62. Robert S. Desowitz, *The Malaria Capers: More Tales of Parasites and People, Research and Reality* (New York: W.W. Norton, 1991), 230.

63. Hart, "Southwest Pacific Area," 578.

64. Condon-Rall, "Allied Cooperation in Malaria Prevention and Control."

65. Condon-Rall, "Allied Cooperation in Malaria Prevention and Control."

66. Hart, "Southwest Pacific Area," 515.

67. Greenwood, "Fight against Malaria."

68. Christine Beadle and Stephen L. Hoffman, "History of Malaria in the United States Naval Forces at War: World War I through the Viet Nam Conflict," *Clinical Infectious Diseases* 16 (February 1993): 320–29.

69. Paul Harper et al., "New Hebrides, Solomon Islands, Saint Matthias Group, and Ryukyu Islands," in *Preventive Medicine in World War II, Volume VI, Communicable Diseases, Malaria*, John Boyd Coates, ed. (Washington, D.C.: Office of the Surgeon General, Department of the Army, 1963), 400.

70. Harper et al., "New Hebrides, Solomon Islands," 433.

71. *Preventive Medicine Manual No. 2 for All Officers*, "Military Control of Malaria and Insect-Borne Diseases," United States Army Forces, Pacific Ocean Areas, Lt. General Robert C. Richardson Jr., Commanding. June 1945.

72. Cowdrey, *Fighting for Life*, 64.

73. Dan Van der Vat, *Pacific Campaign, World War II: The U.S.-Japanese Naval War, 1941–1945* (New York: Simon & Schuster, 1991).

74. Van der Vat, *Pacific Campaign*, 413.

75. Department of the Navy, *The History of the Medical Department of the United States Navy in World War II: A Narrative and Pictorial Volume*, NAVMED P-5031, Vol. 1 (Washington D.C.: Department of the Navy, Bureau of Medicine and Surgery, 1953).

76. Beadle and Hoffman, "History of Malaria in the United States Naval Forces."

77. Joy, "Malaria in American Troops."

78. Paul A. Harper, E. T. Lisansky, and B. E. Sasse, "Malaria and Other Insect Borne Diseases in the South Pacific Campaign, 1942–45, General Aspects and Control Measures," *American Journal of Tropical Medicine* 27 (Supplement 1) (May 1947): 1–67.

79. Russell, "Introduction," 41.

80. Meredith Fischer, "Capturing the Animated Soldier: Private Snafu and the Docile Body Assemblage," *Studies in Popular Culture* 41, no. 1 (Fall 2018): 94–120.

81. W. G. Downs, "Results of an Infantry Regiment of Several Plans of Treatment for *Vivax* Malaria," *American Journal of Tropical Medicine* 26 (January 1946): 67–86.

82. Harper et al., "New Hebrides, Solomon Islands," 429.

83. Joy, "Malaria in American Troops."

84. Weina, "From Atabrine in World War II."

85. Joy, "Malaria in American Troops."

86. Harper et al., "New Hebrides, Solomon Islands," 422–26.

87. Cowdrey, *Fighting for Life*, 180.

88. Harper et al., "New Hebrides, Solomon Islands," 429.

89. Rick Atkinson, *The Day of Battle: The War in Sicily and Italy, 1943–1944* (New York: Henry Holt, 2007), 146.

90. Justin Andrews, "North Africa, Italy, and the Islands of the Mediterranean," in *Preventive Medicine in World War II, Volume VI, Communicable Diseases, Malaria*, John Boyd Coates, ed. (Washington, D.C.: Office of the Surgeon General, Department of the Army, 1963), 263.

91. Russell, "Introduction," 1.

92. *Malaria in the Sicilian Campaign 9 July to 10 September, 1943*, Office of the Surgeon, AFHQ, October 21, 1943.

93. From documents captured by OSS. Cited in Saul Jarcho, "Malaria as a Military Weapon: A Captured German Broadside," *Bulletin of the History of Medicine* 18 (December 1945): 556–59.

94. Myron G. Schultz, "Imported Malaria," *Bulletin of the World Health Organization* 59 (1974): 329–36.

CONCLUSION

1. Albert E. Cowdrey, *The Medic's War: United States Army in the Korean War* (Washington, D.C.: Center of Military History, United States Army, 1987), 54.

2. Ho Wang Lee, "Hemorrhagic Fever with Renal Syndrome in Korea," *Reviews of Infectious Diseases* 11, Supplement 4 (May–June 1989): S846–S876.

3. William S. Mullins, ed., *A Decade of Progress: The United States Army Medical Department, 1959–1969* (Washington, D.C.: Office of the Surgeon General of the Army, 1971), 31–32.

4. Anthony Fauci, "It Ain't Over Till It's Over: Emerging and Reemerging Infectious Diseases," *New England Journal of Medicine* 387 (December 1, 2022): 2009–10.

BIBLIOGRAPHY

BOOKS

Adams, George Worthington. *Doctors in Blue: The Medical History of the Union Army in the Civil War*. Baton Rouge: Louisiana State University Press, 1952.

Altman, Lawrence. *Who Goes First: The Story of Self-Experimentation in Medicine*. New York: Random House, 1986.

Anderson, Robert, ed. *Preventive Medicine in World War II: Special Fields*. Washington, D.C.: Office of the Surgeon General, Department of the Army, 1969.

Ashburn, P. M. *The Elements of Military Hygiene Especially Arranged for Officers and Men of the Line*. Boston: Houghton Mifflin Company, 1909.

———. *A History of the Medical Department of the United States Army*. Boston: Houghton Mifflin Company, 1929.

Atkinson, Rick. *The Day of Battle: The War in Sicily and Italy, 1943–1944*. New York: Henry Holt, 2007.

Barnes, Joseph. *Medical and Surgical History of the War of the Rebellion, Medical Volume, Part 1*. Washington, D.C.: Government Printing Office, 1870.

Barry, John. *The Great Influenza: The Epic Story of the Deadliest Plague in History*. New York: Penguin Books, 2004.

Bayne-Jones, Stanhope. *The Evolution of Preventive Medicine in the United States Army, 1607–1939*. Washington, D.C.: Office of the Surgeon General, Department of the Army, 1968.

Beall, Otho, and Richard Shryock. *Cotton Mather: First Significant Figure in American Medicine*. Baltimore: Johns Hopkins University Press, 1954.

Bean, William. *Walter Reed: A Biography*. Charlottesville: University Press of Virginia, 1982.

Binger, Carl. *Revolutionary Doctor: Benjamin Rush, 1746–1813*. New York: W. W. Norton, 1966.

Bollet, Alfred Jay. *Civil War Medicine: Challenges and Triumphs*. Tucson, AZ: Galen Press, 2002.

Brooks, Stewart. *Civil War Medicine*. Springfield, IL: Charles C. Thomas, 1966.

Bruno Lina. "History of Pandemics." In *Paleomicrobioilogy*, edited by D. Raoult and M. Drancourt, 199–211. Berlin: Springer-Verlag, 2008.

Byerly, Carol. *Fever of War: The Influenza Epidemic in the U.S. Army during World War I*. New York: New York University Press, 2005.

Carter, H. R. *Some Characteristics of Stegomyia Fasciata Which Affect Its Conveyance of Yellow Fever*. New York: William Wood and Company, 1904.

Cartwright, Frederick F. *Disease and History*. New York: Dorset Press, 1972.

Chambers, Thomas J., and Thomas P. Monath. *The Flaviviruses: Pathogenesis and Immunity*. Amsterdam: Elsevier Academic Press, 2003.

Chisolm, John Julian. *A Manual of Military Surgery for the Use of Surgeons in the Confederate Army with an Appendix of the Rules and Regulations of the Medical Department of the Confederate Army*. Richmond: West & Johnston, 1861. Reprinted by Norman Publishing, 1989.

Cirillo, Vincent J. *Bullets and Bacilli: The Spanish-American War and Military Medicine*. New Brunswick, NJ: Rutgers University Press, 1999.

Coates, John Boyd, ed. *Preventive Medicine in World War II, Volume VI, Communicable Diseases, Malaria*. Washington, D.C.: Office of the Surgeon General, Department of the Army, 1963.

———, ed. *Preventive Medicine in World War II, Volume VII, Communicable Diseases, Arthropodborne Diseases Other Than Malaria*. Washington, D.C.: Office of the Surgeon General, Department of the Army, 1964.

Cowdrey, Albert E. *Fighting for Life: American Military Medicine in World War II*. New York: Free Press, 1994.

———. *The Medic's War: United States Army in the Korean War*. Washington, D.C.: Center of Military History, United States Army, 1987.

Crosby, Alfred. *America's Forgotten Pandemic: The Influenza of 1918*. Cambridge: Cambridge University Press, 2003.

———. *Epidemic and Peace*. Westport, CT: Greenwood Press, 1976.

Crosby, Molly Caldwell. *The American Plague: The Untold Story of Yellow Fever, the Epidemic That Shaped Our History*. New York: Berkley Books, 2006.

Cunningham, H. H. *Doctors in Gray: The Confederate Medical Service*. Baton Rouge: Louisiana State University Press, 1958.

Cushing, Harvey. *The Life of Sir William Osler*. Oxford: Clarendon Press, 1926.

Davis, William C. *The Imperiled Union: Volume One, The Deep Waters of the Proud*. Garden City, NJ: Doubleday, 1982.

Delaporte, Francois. *The History of Yellow Fever: An Essay on the Birth of Tropical Medicine*. Cambridge, MA: MIT Press, 1991.

Denny, Robert. *Civil War Medicine: Care and Comfort of the Wounded*. New York: Sterling Publishing, 1995.

Department of the Navy. *The History of the Medical Department of the United States Navy in World War II: A Narrative and Pictorial Volume, NAVMED*

P-5031, Vol. 1. Washington, D.C.: Department of the Navy, Bureau of Medicine and Surgery, 1953.

Desowitz, Robert S. *The Malaria Capers: More Tales of Parasites and People, Research and Reality.* New York: W. W. Norton, 1991.

Duffy, John. *Epidemics in Colonial America.* Baton Rouge: Louisiana State University Press, 1953.

Eshner, Augustus. *Fevers: Including General Considerations, Typhoid Fever, Typhus Fever, Influenza, Malarial Fever, Yellow Fever, Variola, Relapsing Fever, Weil's Disease, Thermic Fever, Dengue, Miliary Fever, Mountain Fever, etc.* London: F. A. Davis Publishers, 1895.

Espinosa, Mariola. *Epidemic Invasions: Yellow Fever and the Limits of Cuban Independence, 1878–1930.* Chicago: University of Chicago Press, 2009.

Fenn, Elizabeth. *Pox Americana: The Great Smallpox Epidemic of 1775–1782.* New York: Hill and Wang, 2001.

Flexner, James Thomas. *George Washington in the American Revolution (1775–1783).* Boston: Little, Brown and Company, 1967.

Foote, Shelby. *The Civil War, a Narrative: Fort Sumter to Perryville.* New York: Random House, 1958.

Freemon, Frank. *Gangrene and Glory: Medical Care during the American Civil War.* Urbana: University of Illinois Press, 2001.

———. *Microbes and Minie Balls: An Annotated Bibliography of Civil War Medicine.* Rutherford: Associated University Presses, 1993.

Gianella, Ralph A. "Salmonella," in Samuel Baron, ed., *Medical Microbiology*, 4th ed. Galveston: University of Texas Medical Branch. Accessed November 21, 2021. https://www.ncbi.nlm.nih.gov/books/NBK7627/.

Gibson, John M. *Soldier in White: The Life of General George Miller Sternberg.* Durham, N.C.: Duke University Press, 1958.

Gillett, Mary. *The Army Medical Department: 1775–1818.* Washington, D.C.: Center of Military History, United States Army, 1981.

———. *The Army Medical Department: 1818–1865.* Washington, D.C.: Center of Military History, United States Army, 1987.

———. *The Army Medical Department: 1917–1941.* Washington, D.C.: Center of Military History, United States Army, 2009.

Greene, H. Leon. *The Confederate Yellow Fever Conspiracy: The Germ Warfare Plot of Luke Pryor Blackburn, 1864–1865.* Jefferson, NC: McFarland , 2019.

Gross, Samuel David. *A Manual of Military Surgery of Hints on the Emergencies of Field, Camp and Hospital Practice.* Philadelphia: Lippincott, 1861. Reprinted by Norman Publishing, 1988.

Hamilton, Frank Hastings. *A Practical Treatise on Military Surgery.* New York: Balliere Brothers, 1861. Reprinted by Norman Publishing, 1989.

Henry, J. J. *Arnold's Campaign against Canada*. Albany, NY: Joel Munsell, 1877.

Hoehling, A. A. *The Great Epidemic*. Boston: Little, Brown and Company, 1961.

Ireland, Merrit. *Medical Department of the United States Army in the World War*. Vol. 9, *Communicable Diseases*. Washington, D.C.: U.S. Army, 1929.

Kelly, Howard A. *Walter Reed and Yellow Fever*. Baltimore: Medical Standard Book Company, 1906.

Kolata, Gina. *Influenza: The Story of the Great Influenza Pandemic of 1918 and the Search for the Virus That Caused It*. New York: Farrar, Straus and Giroux, 1999.

Kotar, S. L., and J. E. Gessler. *Yellow Fever: A Worldwide History*. Jefferson, NC: McFarland, 2017.

LaRoche, D. *Yellow Fever, Considered in Its Historical, Pathological, Etiological, and Therapeutic Relations*. Vol. 2. Philadelphia: Blanchard and Lea, 1855.

Levine, Arnold. *Viruses*. New York: Scientific American Library, 1992.

Liddell Hart, B. H. *The Real War:1914–1918*. London: Little, Brown and Company, 1930.

Longstreet, James. *From Manassas to Appomattox: Memoirs of the Civil War in America*. Secaucas, NJ: Blue and Grey Press, 1984.

Matloff, Maurice, and Edwin M. Snell. *Strategic Planning for Coalition Warfare, 1942–1943*. Washington, D.C.: Office of the Chief of Military History, 1953.

McCallum, Jack. *Leonard Wood: Rough Rider, Surgeon, Architect of American Imperialism*. New York: New York University Press, 2006.

McCullough, David. *The Path between the Seas: The Creation of the Panama Canal, 1870–1914*. New York: Simon and Schuster, 1977.

McDonald, Lyn. *The Roses of No Man's Land*. New York: Atheneum, 1980.

McPherson, James M. *Battle Cry of Freedom: The Civil War Era*. New York: Oxford University Press, 1988.

Middlekauff, Robert. *The Glorious Cause: The American Revolution, 1763–1789*. New York: Oxford University Press, 1982.

Moore, Samuel Preston. *A Manual of Military Surgery Prepared for the Use of the Confederate States Army*. Richmond: Ayres & Wade, 1863. Reprinted by Norman Publishing, 1989.

Mullins, William S., ed. *A Decade of Progress: The United States Army Medical Department, 1959–1969*. Washington, D.C.: Office of the Surgeon General of the Army, 1971.

Nevins, Allan. *The War for the Union: The Improvised War, 1861–1862*. New York: Charles Scribner's Sons, 1959.

———. *The War for the Union: War Becomes Revolution, 1862–1863*. New York: Charles Scribner's Sons, 1960.

Oaks, Stanley, Violane Mitchell, Greg Pearson, and Charles Carpenter, eds. *Malaria: Obstacles and Opportunities*. Washington, D.C.: National Academy Press, 1991.

Osler, William. *The Principles and Practice of Medicine Designed for the Use of Practitioners and Students of Medicine*. New York: D. Appleton and Company, 1899.

Owen, William O. *The Medical Department of the United States Army during the Period of the Revolution (1776–1786)*. New York: Paul B. Hoeber, 1920.

Packard, Francis R. *History of Medicine in the United States*. Vol. 1. New York: Paul B. Hoeber, 1931.

Packard, Randall. *The Making of a Tropical Disease: A Short History of Malaria*. Baltimore: Johns Hopkins University Press, 2007.

Petit, Dorothy Ann, and Janice Bailie. *A Cruel Wind: American Experiences in the Pandemic Influenza; 1918–1920, A Social History*. Murfreesboro, TN: Timberlane Books, 2008.

Pierce, John, and Jim Writer. *Yellow Jack: How Yellow Fever Ravaged America and Walter Reed Discovered Its Deadly Secrets*. Hoboken, NJ: Wiley, 2005.

Price-Smith, Andrew T. *Contagion and Chaos: Disease, Ecology, and National Security in the Era of Globalization*. Cambridge, MA: MIT Press, 2009.

Prinzing, Friedrich. *Epidemics Resulting from Wars*. Oxford: Clarendon Press, 1916.

Raoult, D., and M. Drancourt, eds. *Paleomicrobioilogy*. Berlin: Springer-Verlag, 2008.

Reed, Walter, James Carroll, A. Agramonte, and Jesse W. Lazear. *The Etiology of Yellow Fever—A Preliminary Note*. Columbus, OH: Berlin Printing Company, 1901.

Reiss, Oscar. *Medicine and the American Revolution*. Jefferson, NC: McFarland, 1998.

Romaine, Benjamin. *Observations, Reasons and Facts Disproving Importation and Also All Specific Personal Contagion in Yellow Fever from Any Local Origin, and That Which Arises from the Common Changes of the Atmosphere*. New York: J. C. Spear, 1823.

Sanchez, J. L. *Carlos Finlay: His Life and Work*. Havana, Cuba: Editorial José Marti, 1999.

Seaman, Rebecca, ed. *Epidemics and War: The Impact of Disease on Major Conflicts in History*. Santa Barbara, CA: ABC-CLIO, 2018.

Smallman-Raynor, M. R., and A. D. Cliff. *War Epidemics: An Historical Geography of Infectious Diseases in Military Conflict and Civil Strife, 1850–2000*. Oxford: Oxford University Press, 2006.

Smart, Charles. *Medical and Surgical History of the War of the Rebellion, Medical Volume, Third Part*. Washington, D.C.: Government Printing Office, 1888.

Snowden, Frank. *The Conquest of Malaria: Italy, 1900–1962*. New Haven, CT: Yale University Press, 2006.

———. *Epidemics and Society: From the Black Death to the Present*. New Haven, CT: Yale University Press, 2020.

Spector, Ronald H. *Eagle against the Sun: The American War with Japan*. New York: Free Press, 1985.

Spinney, Laura. *Pale Rider: The Spanish Influenza of 1918 and How It Changed the World*. New York: Public Affairs, 1917.

Steiner, Paul. *Disease in the Civil War: National Biological Warfare in 1861–1865*. Springfield, IL: Charles C. Thomas, 1968.

Sternberg, George M. *A Manual of Bacteriology*. New York: William Wood, 1892.

———. *Report on the Etiology and Prevention of Yellow Fever*. Washington, D.C.: Government Printing Office, 1890.

Sternberg, Martha. *George Miller Sternberg: A Biography*. Chicago: American Medical Association, 1920.

Steward, H. D. *Recollections of a Regimental Medical Officer*. Melbourne: Melbourne University Press, 1983.

Touatre, Just. *Yellow Fever: Clinical Notes*. New Orleans: New Orleans Medical and Surgical Journal, 1898.

Tregaskis, Richard. *Guadalcanal Diary*. New York: Random House, 1943.

Tripler, Charles Stuart, and George Curtis Blackman. *Hand-book for the Military Surgeon*. Cincinnati, OH: R. Clarke, 1861. Reprinted by Norman Publishing, 1989.

Truby, Albert. *Memoir of Walter Reed: The Yellow Fever Episode*. New York: Paul B. Hoeber, 1943.

Vainio, Jari, and Felicity Cutts. "Yellow Fever," from *World Health Organization. Division of Emerging and Other Communicable Diseases Surveillance and Control*. Geneva, 1998.

Van der Vatr, Dan. *The Pacific Campaign, World War II: The U.S.-Japanese Naval War, 1941–1945*. New York: Simon & Schuster, 1991.

Watts, Sheldon. *Epidemics and History: Disease, Power and Imperialism*. New Haven, CT: Yale University Press, 1997.

Williams, Tony. *The Pox and the Covenant: Mather, Franklin, and the Epidemic That Changed America's Destiny*. Naperville, IL: Sourcebooks, 2010.

Willmott, H. P. *Empires in the Balance: Japanese and Allied Pacific Strategies to April 1942*. Annapolis: Naval Institute Press, 1982.

Wilson, James C., et al. *Fevers including General Considerations, Typhoid Fever, Yellow Fever, Variola, Relapsing Fever, Weil's Disease, Thermic Fever, Dengue, Miliary Fever, Mountain Fever, etc.* London: F. A. Davis Publishers, 1895.

Wood, L. N. *Walter Reed: Doctor in Uniform*. New York: Julian Messner, 1943.

Woodbridge, John Eliot. *Typhoid Fever and Its Abortive Treatment*. Cleveland, OH: L. Leavengood, 1896.

Woodward, Joseph Janvier. *Outlines of the Chief Camp Diseases of the United States Armies as Observed during the Present War*. Philadelphia: Lippincott, 1863. Reprinted San Francisco: Norman Publishing, 1992.

Wyman, Walter. *Yellow Fever: Its Nature, Diagnosis, Treatment, and Prophylaxis and Quarantine Regulations Relating Thereto*. Washington, D.C.: Government Printing Office, 1899.

Zabecki, David. *The German 1918 Offensives: A Case Study in the Operational Level of War*. London: Routledge, 2006.

Zinsser, Hans. *Rats, Lice, and History: Being a Study in Biography, Which, after Twelve Preliminary Chapters Indispensable for the Preparation of the Lay Reader, Deals with the Life History of Typhus Fever*. Boston: Little, Brown and Company, 1934.

ARTICLES

Alexander, J. Browning. "Cases Resembling Encephalitis Lethargica: Occurring during the Influenza Epidemic." *British Medical Journal* 1 (June 28, 1919): 794–95.

Agramonte, Aristedes. "The Inside History of a Great Medical Discovery." *Scientific Monthly* 1 (1915): 209–37.

Artenstein, Andrew, et al. "History of U.S. Military Contributions to the Study of Vaccines against Infectious Diseases." *Military Medicine* 170 (April Supplement 2005): 3–11.

Baker, Henry. "The Etiology and Pathology of Typhoid Fever." Reprinted from *Annual Report of the Michigan State Board of Health for the Year 1886*. Accessed November 15, 2021. https://collections.nlm.nih.gov/bookviewer ?PID=nlmnlmuid-10151430-bk.

Balikagala, B., et al. "Evidence of Artemisinin-Resistant Malaria in Africa." *New England Journal of Medicine* 385 (September 23, 2021): 1163–71.

Barnes, Joseph K. "The Annual Report of the Surgeon General." *Medical and Surgical Reporter* 16 (1867): 75–77.

Barr, Justin, and Scott Podolsky. "A National Medical Response to Crisis—The Legacy of World War II." *New England Journal of Medicine* 383 (August 13, 2020): 613–15.

Beadle, Christine, and Stephen L. Hoffman. "History of Malaria in the United States Naval Forces at War: World War I through the Viet Nam Conflict." *Clinical Infectious Diseases* 16 (February 1993): 320–29.

Bean, William B. "Walter Reed and the Ordeal of Human Experiments." *Bulletin of the History of Medicine* 51 (Spring 1977): 75–92.

Becker, Alexander. "Typhoid Fever: Its Causes and Sources as Explained by the Germ Theory of Disease." Reprinted from *Boston Medical and Surgical Journal*, 1879. Accessed November 15, 2021. https://collections.nlm.nih.gov /bookviewer?PID=nlm:nlmuid-101683349-bk.

Becker, Ann M. "Smallpox at the Siege of Boston: 'Vigilance against This Most Dangerous Enemy,'" *Historical Journal of Massachusetts* 45 (2017): 43–75.

Benenson, Abram. "Immunization and Military Medicine." *Reviews of Infectious Disease* 6 (January–February 1984): 1–12.

Bhandari, Jenish, Pawan Theda, and Elizabeth DeVos. "Typhoid Fever." Accessed February 23, 2021. www.ncbi.nlm.nih.gov/books/NBK 5575131/.

Blake, John. "Smallpox Inoculation in Colonial Boston." *Journal of the History of Medicine and the Allied Sciences* 8 (1953): 283–300.

Blanco, Richard. "Military Medicine in Northern New York, 1776–1777." *New York History* 63 (1982): 39–58.

Bloomfield, Arthur L. "A Bibliography of Internal Medicine: Yellow Fever." *Bulletin of the History of Medicine* 30 (May–June 1956): 213–32.

Boylston, Arthur. "Daniel Sutton, a Forgotten 18th century Clinical Scientist." *Journal of the Royal Society of Medicine* 105 (February 2012): 85–87.

Brieman, Joel, and D. A. Henderson. "Diagnosis and Management of Smallpox." *New England Journal of Medicine* 346 (April 25, 2002): 1300–307.

Broad, William J., and Judith Miller. "Report Provides New Details of Soviet Smallpox Accident." *New York Times*, June 15, 2002.

Byerly, Carol. "The U.S. Military and the Influenza Pandemic of 1918–19." *Public Health Reports* 125 (April 2010); *Supplement 3: The 1918–1919 Influenza Pandemic in the United States* (April 2010): 82–91.

Caillé, Augusto. "Our Present Knowledge Concerning the Aetiology of Typhoid Fever." *New York Medical Journal* (January 19, 1889). Reprint. Accessed November 17, 2021. https://collections.nlm.nih.gov/bookviewer?PID=nlm: nlmuid-101723401-bk.

Carroll, James. "Remarks on the History, Cause, and Mode of Transmission of Yellow Fever and the Occurrence of Similar Types of Fatal Fevers in Places Where Yellow Fever Is Not Known to Have Existed." Reprinted from *Journal of the Association of Military Surgeons of the United States*, Carlisle, PA: Association of Military Surgeons, 1903.

Centers for Disease Control and Prevention. "Control of Infectious Diseases, 1900–1999." *Journal of the American Medical Association* 282 (1999): 1029–32.

Chaves-Carballo, Enrique. "Carlos Finlay and Yellow Fever: Triumph over Adversity." *Military Medicine* 10 (2005): 881–85.

Chertow, Daniel S., et al. "Influenza Circulation in United States Army Training Camps before and during the 1918 Influenza Pandemic: Clues to Early

Detection of Pandemic Viral Emergence." *Public Health Reports* 125, Supplement 3 (2015): 6–8.

Cirillo, Vincent. "Fever and Reform: The Typhoid Epidemic in the Spanish-American War." *Journal of the History of Medicine and Allied Sciences* 55 (October 2000): 363–97.

———. "'The Patriotic Order': Sanitation and Typhoid Fever in the National Encampments during the Spanish-American War." *Army History* 49 (2000): 17–23.

Comfort, Nathaniel. "The Prisoner as Model Organism: Malaria Research at Stateville Penitentiary." *Studies in History, Philosophy, Biology, and Biomedical Science* 40 (September 2009): 190–203.

Condon-Rall, Mary Ellen. "Allied Cooperation in Malaria Prevention and Control: The World War II Southwest Pacific Experience." *Journal of the History of Medicine and Allied Sciences* 46 (October 1991): 493–513.

Coombs, Howard G. "The Influenza Pandemic of 1918: Military Observations for Today from COVID-19." In *COVID-19: NATO in the Age of Pandemics*, Thierry Tardy, ed. NATO Defense College. Accessed April 8, 2021. https://www.ndc.nato.int/news/news.php?icode=1440.

Cooper, W. Clark. "Summary of Anti-Malarial Drugs." *Public Health Reports* 64 (June 10, 1949): 717–32.

Corbin, H. C., and G. M. Magruder. "Report of Passed Assistant Surgeon Magruder on the Work Done at Montauk Point." *Public Health Reports (1896–1970)* 14 (1899): 149–52.

Councell, Clara E. "War and Infectious Disease." *Public Health Reports* 56 (March, 21, 1941): 547–73.

Creighton, C. "The Origin of Yellow Fever." *North American Review* 139 (October 1884): 335–47.

Cunha, Burke A. "Influenza: Historical Aspects of Epidemics and Pandemics." *Infectious Disease Clinics of North America* 18 (2004): 141–55.

Deist, Wilhelm, and E. J. Feuchtwanger. "The Military Collapse of the German Empire: The Reality behind the Stab-in-the-Back Myth." *War in History* 3 (April 1996): 186–207.

Del Regato, Juan A. "Carlos Juan Finlay (1833-1915)." *Journal of Public Health Policy* 22, no. 1 (2001): 98–104.

Doty, Alvah H. "The Scientific Prevention of Yellow Fever." *North American Review* 167 (1898): 681–89.

Downs, W. G. "Results of an Infantry Regiment of Several Plans of Treatment for Vivax Malaria." *American Journal of Tropical Medicine* 26 (January 1946): 67–86.

Eager, J. M. "The Early History of Quarantine: Origin of Sanitary Measures Directed against Yellow Fever." *Yellow Fever Institute Bulletin* 12 (March 1903): 3–27.

Espinosa, Mariola. "The Question of Racial Immunity to Yellow Fever in History and Historiography." *Social Science History* 38 (Fall/Winter 2014): 437–53.

———. "The Threat from Havana: Southern Public Health, Yellow Fever, and the U.S. Intervention in the Cuban Struggle for Independence, 1878–1898." *Journal of Southern History* 72 (2006): 541–68.

Eyler, John. "The Fog of Research: Influenza Vaccine Trials during the 1918–19 Pandemic." *Journal of the History of Medicine and the Allied Sciences* 64 (October 2009): 401–28.

Fairley, N. H. "Researches in Paludine (M.4888) in Malaria." *Transactions of the Royal Society of Tropical Medicine and Hygiene* 40 (October 1946): 105–51.

Fargey, Kathleen. "The Deadliest Enemy." *Army History* 111 (Spring 2019): 24–39.

Faulkner, Edgar. "Disappearing Doughboys: The American Expeditionary Force's Straggler Crisis in the Meuse-Argonne." *Army History* 4 (Spring 2012): 7–25.

Finlay, C. E. "Carlos Finlay and Yellow Fever." *Journal of Parasitology* 28 (April 1942): 172–74.

Fischer, Meredith. "Capturing the Animated Soldier: Private Snafu and the Docile Body Assemblage." *Studies in Popular Culture* 41 (Fall 2018): 94–120.

Fletcher, Willian, and K. Kanagarayer. "Plasmochin in the Treatment of Malaria." *Indian Medical Gazette* 62 (1927): 499–506.

Freeborn, Stanley B. "Problems Created by Returning Malaria Carriers." *Public Health Reports* 59 (March 17, 1944): 357–63.

Geissler, Erhard. "German Flooding of the Pontine Marshes in World War II: Biological Warfare or Total War Tactic?" *Politics and the Life Sciences* 29 (March 2010): 2–23.

Gibbons, Robert V., Matthew Streitz, Tatyana Babina, and Jessica Fried. "Dengue and U.S. Military Operations from Spanish-American War through Today." *Emerging Infectious Diseases Journal* 18 (April 2012). Accessed January 1, 2022. https://www.ncf.cdc.gov/eid/article/18/4/11–0134_article.

Gibbs Mark J., John S. Armstrong, and Adrian J. Gibbs. "The Haemagglutinin Gene, but Not the Neuraminidase Gene of 'Spanish Flu' Was a Recombinant." *Philosophical Transactions: Biological Sciences* 356 (December 2001): 1845–1855.

Girard, Philippe R. "Liberté, Egalité, Esclavage: French Revolutionary Ideals and the Failure of the Leclerc Expedition to Saint-Domingue." *French Colonial History* 6 (2005): 55–77.

Greenwood, John T. "The Fight against Malaria in the Papua and New Guinea Campaigns." *Army History* 59 (Summer–Fall 2003): 16–28.

Grist, N. R. "Pandemic Influenza." *British Medical Journal* 2 (December 1979): 1632.

Groschel, Dieter, and Richard B. Hornick. "Who Introduced Typhoid Vaccination: Almroth Wright or Richard Pfeiffer?" *Review of Infectious Diseases* 3 (1981): 1251–1254.

Hammond, William A. "Annual Report of the Surgeon General, U.S.A." *Boston Medical and Surgical Journal* 67 (1863): 437–43.

Harcourt, Bernard E. "Making Willing Bodies: The University of Chicago Human Experiments at Stateville Penitentiary." *Social Research* 78 (Summer 2011): 443–78.

Harper, Paul A., E. T. Lisansky, and B. E. Sasse. "Malaria and Other Insect Borne Diseases in the South Pacific Campaign, 1942–45, General Aspects and Control Measures." *American Journal of Tropical Medicine* 27 (Supplement 1) (May 1947): 1–67.

Hirsch, Edwin F., and Marion McKinney. "Further Studies on the Influenza Epidemic at Camp Grant." *Journal of Infectious Diseases* 25 (November 1919): 394–98.

Hollenbeck, James E. "The 1918–1919 Influenza Pandemic: A Pale Horse Rides Home from War." *Bios* 1 (March 2002): 19–27.

Hubbard, George H. "Spurious Vaccination: Inoculation with Virus Supposed to Be Syphilitic." *Medical and Surgical Reporter* 14 (1866): 103.

Humphries, Mark Osborne. "Paths of Infection: The First World War and the Origins of the 1918 Influenza Pandemic." *War in History* 1 (2014): 55–81.

Humphreys, Margaret. "The Influenza of 1918: Evolutionary Perspectives in a Historical Context." *Evolution, Medicine, and Public Health* (2018): 219–29.

Influenza Committee of the Advisory Board. "A Report on the Influenza Epidemic in the British Armies in France, 1918." *British Medical Journal* 2 (November 9, 1918): 505–509. Accessed January 6, 2021. Reprint https://collections.nlm.nih.gov/bookviewer?PID=nlm;nlmuid-101473324-bk.

Jackson, Henry. "A Review of the Diseases Contracted in the Cuban Campaign of 1898." *The Medical and Surgical Reports of the Boston City Hospital, Tenth Series,* 1899. From reprint. Accessed November 19, 2021. https://collections.nlm.nih.gov/bookviewer?PID=nlm;nlmuid-101597722-bk.

Jarcho, Saul. "Malaria as a Military Weapon: A Captured German Broadside." *Bulletin of the History of Medicine* 18 (December 1945): 556–59.

Jefferson, Tom, and Eliana Ferroni. "The Spanish Flu through the BMJ's Eyes." *British Medical Journal* 339 (December 2009): 19–26.

Jordan, Edwin O. "Observations on the Bacteriology of Influenza." *Journal of Infectious Diseases* 25 (July 1919): 28–40.

Joy, Robert J. T. "Malaria in American Troops in the South and Southwest Pacific in World War II." *Medical History* 43 (1999): 192–207.

Katz, Robert S. "Influenza 1918–1919: A Study in Mortality." *Bulletin of the History of Medicine* 48 (Fall 1974): 416–22.

Kelly, Howard A. "James Carroll 1854–1907." *Proceedings of the Washington Academy of Sciences* (1980): 204–207.

Kelvin, K. W., and Kwok-Yung Yuen. "In Memory of Patrick Manson, Founding Father of Tropical Medicine and the Discovery of Vector-Borne Infections." *Emerging Microbes and Infections* (2012). Accessed July 14, 2021. www.ncbi .nlm.nih.gov/PMC3630944/pdf/emi201232a.pdf.

Kenyon, Georgina. "Australian Army Infected Troops and Internees in Second World War." *British Medical Journal* 318 (May 1999): 1233.

Kolakowski, Christopher L. "Gallantry, Courage, and Devotion to Duty." *Army History* 116 (Summer 2020): 6–23.

Kolata, Gina. "Genetic Material of Virus from 1918 Flu Is Found." *New York Times*, March 21, 1997.

Lacey, John. "Memoirs." *Pennsylvania Magazine of Historical Biography* 25 (1901): 203–204.

Langford, Christopher. "Did the 1918–19 Influenza Pandemic Originate in China?" *Population and Development Review* 31 (2005): 473–505.

Laurence, William L. "New Drugs to Combat Malaria Are Tested in Prisons for Army." *New York Times*, March 5, 1945.

Lee, Ho Wang. "Hemorrhagic Fever with Renal Syndrome in Korea." *Reviews of Infectious Diseases* 11, Supplement 4 (May–June 1989): S846–S876.

Leishman, W. B. "Vaccines for Influenza." *British Medical Journal* 2 (October 26, 1918): 470.

Lumsden, I. L. "Influenza: Avoid It and Prevent Its Spread." *Public Health Reports (1896–1970)* 33 (October 1918): 731–32.

Markel, Howard. "Dr. Osler's Relapsing Fever." *Journal of the American Medical Association* 295 (2006): 2886–87.

Mayo Clinic. "Typhoid Fever." Accessed November 23, 2021. https://www.mayocli nic.org/diseases-conditions/typhoid-fever/symptoms-causes/syc-20378661.

McGrath, Nick. "Fort Devens Massachusetts." *On Point* 20 (2015): 44–47.

McNeill, J. R. "Yellow Jack and Geopolitics: Environment, Epidemics, and the Struggles for Empire in the American Tropics, 1640–1830." *Review Fernand Braudel Center No. 4, The Environment and World History* 4 (2004): 343–64.

Medical Research Council Committee on Malaria. "Mepacrine for Malaria." *British Medical Journal* 2 (November 18, 1944): 664.

Mehra, Akhil. "Politics of Participation: Walter Reed's Yellow Fever Experiments." *American Medical Association Journal of Ethics* 11 (2009): 326–30.

Miller, Robert I. "The Impact of Quarantine on Military Operations." Maxwell Air Force Base, AL: Air University, 2005.

Monath, Thomas P. "Yellow Fever: An Update." *Lancet Infectious Diseases* 1 (2001): 11–20.

Moran, John. "Mosquitoes and Yellow Fever." *British Medical Journal* 1 (1901): 1102.

Morens, David, and Jeffery Taubenberger. "Predominant Role of Bacterial Pneumonia as a Cause of Death in Pandemic Influenza: Implications for Pandemic Influenza Preparedness." *Journal of Infectious Diseases* 198 (2008): 962–70.

Morrison, David. "Pandemics and National Security." *Great Decisions* (2006): 93–102.

Morse, Stephen. "Influenza: Studying the Lessons of History." *Proceedings of the National Academy of Sciences of the United States of America* 104 (May 2007): 7313–14.

Mortimer, P. P. "Was Encephalitis Lethargica a Post-Influenzal or Some Other Phenomenon? Time to Re-Examine the Problem." *Epidemiology and Infection* 137 (April 2009): 449–55.

Navarro, Julian. "Influenza in 1918: An Epidemic in Images." *Public Health Reports Supplement 3* 125 (2010): 9–14.

"Obituary, Surgeon General Walter Wyman." *Military Surgeon* 29 (December 1911): 699.

Osler, William. "Discussion of G. M. Sternberg, 'The Bacillus Icteroides (Sanarelli) and Bacillus x (Sternberg).'" *Transactions of the Association of American Physicians* 13 (1898): 71.

———. "The Study of Fevers in the South." *Journal of the American Medical Association* 26 (1896): 999–1004.

Oxford, J. S. "The So-Called Great Spanish Influenza Pandemic of 1918 May Have Originated in France in 1916." *Philosophical Transactions: Biological Sciences* 356 (December 2001): 1857–59.

———. "World War I May Have Allowed the Emergence of 'Spanish' Influenza." *Lancet: Infectious Diseases* 2, no. 2 (2002): 111–14.

Paltzer, Seth. "The Other Foe: The U.S. Army's Fight against Malaria in the Pacific Theater, 1942–1945." *Army History* (Winter 2016): 6–12.

Patterson, K. David, and Gerald Pyle. "The Geography and Mortality of the 1918 Influenza Pandemic." *Bulletin of the History of Medicine* 65 (Spring 1991): 4–21.

Peller, Sigismund. "Walter Reed, C. Finlay, and Their Predecessors around 1800." *Bulletin of the History of Medicine* 33 (May–June 1959): 195–211.

Person, Gustav. "The Flu Strikes Belvoir: Camp A. A. Humphreys and the Spanish Influenza Pandemic of 1918." *On Point* 14 (Fall 2008): 8–13.

Pierce, John R. "In the Interest of Humanity and the Cause of Science: The Yellow Fever Volunteers." *Military Medicine* 168 (November 2003): 857–63.

Preston, Richard. "The Demon in the Freezer: How Smallpox, a Disease Officially Eradicated Twenty Years Ago, Became the Biggest Bioterrorist Threat We Now Face." *New Yorker*, July 12, 1999, 47–61.

Proust and Wurtz. "Yellow Fever." *Public Health Reports* 15 (September 7, 1900): 2197–202.

Rafuse, Ethan. "Typhoid and Tumult: Lincoln's Response to General McClellan's Bout with Typhoid Fever." *Journal of the Abraham Lincoln Association* 18, no. 2 (1997): 1–16.

Reed, Walter. "Recent Researches Concerning the Etiology, Propagation, and Prevention of Yellow Fever, by the United States Army Commission." *Journal of Hygiene* 2 (April 1902): 101–19.

Reidel, Stefan. "Edward Jenner and the History of Smallpox and Vaccination." *Baylor University Medical Center Proceedings* 18 (2005): 21–25.

Rivers, Thomas M. "Epidemic Diseases." *Proceedings of the American Philosophical Society* 91 (February 1947): 88–94.

Ross, Ronald. "William Crawford Gorgas." *Science Progress in the Twentieth Century (1919–1933)* 15 (January 1921): 452–55.

Rostker, Bernard. "Providing for Casualties of War." In *The American Experience in World War II*. Santa Monica, CA: RAND Corporation. Accessed June 2, 2021. https://www.jstor/stable/10.7249/j.ctt2tt90p.17.

Royal College of Physicians. "Prevention and Treatment of Influenza." *British Medical Journal* 2 (November 16, 1918): 546.

Rozo, Michelle, and Gigi Kwik Gronvall. "The Reemergent 1977 H1 N1 Strain and the Gain-of-Function Debate." *mBio*. Accessed May 3, 2021. https://journals.asm.org/doi/10.1128/mBio.01013-15.

Salmi, Derek M. "Slim's Burma Campaign." Air University Press. Accessed June 1, 2021. http://www.jstor.com/stable/resrep13911.9.

"Salmonella Infections." *British Medical Journal* 1 (March 1945): 451–52.

Sanchez, Jose. "Influenza in the U.S. Military: An Overview." *Journal of Infectious Diseases and Treatment* 2 (2016): 1–7.

Sargeant, Howland, and Henrietta Creamer. "Enemy Patents." *Law and Contemporary Problems, Vol. 1: Enemy Property* 11 (1945): 92–108.

Sartin, Jeffrey S. "Infectious Diseases during the Civil War: The Triumph of the 'Third Army.'" *Clinical Infectious Diseases* 16 (April 1993): 580–84.

Schultz, Myron G. "Imported Malaria." *Bulletin of the World Health Organization*, 59 (1974): 329–36.

Shanks, George Dennis. "Decreased Mortality of Falciparum Malaria in Anemic Prisoners of War?" *American Journal of Tropical Medicine and Hygiene* 6 (December 2020): 2171–73.

———. "Malaria-Associated Mortality in Australian and British Prisoners of War on the Thai-Burma Railway, 1943–1944." *American Journal of Tropical Medicine and Hygiene* 100 (2019): 846–50.

Shanks, G. D., G. J. Milinovich, M. Waller, and A. C. A. Clements. "Spatio-Temporal Investigation of the 1918 Influenza Pandemic in Military Populations Indicates Two Different Viruses." *Epidemiology and Infection* 143 (July 2015): 1816–25.

Shryock, Richard. "A Medical Prospective on the Civil War." *American Quarterly* 14 (1962): 161–73.

Sinton, J. A. "Malaria in War." *Ulster Medical Journal* 15 (1946): 3–28.

Smallman-Raynor, Matthew, and Andrew D. Clift. "Epidemic Diffusion Processes in a System of U.S. Military Camps: Transfer Diffusion and the Spread of Typhoid Fever in the Spanish-American War, 1898." *Annals of the Association of American Geographers* 91 (2001): 71–91.

Smith, Arthur M., and Craig Hooper. "The Mosquito Can Be More Dangerous Than the Mortar Round: The Obligations of Command." *Naval War College Review* 58 (Winter 2005): 77–87.

Smith, Dale C. "The Rise and Fall of Typho-Malarial Fever: I. Origins." *Journal of the History of Medicine and Allied Sciences* 37, no. 3 (April 1982): 182–220.

Sohn, Kyongsei, and Bryan L. Boulier. "Estimating Parameters of the 1918–1919 Influenza Epidemic on U.S. Military Bases." College at Brockport: State University of New York. Accessed February 20, 2021. https://digtitalcommons.brockport.edu/bus_facpub/20.

Soper, George. "The Influenza Pandemic in the American Army Camps during September and October 1918." *Science, New Series* 48 (November 8, 1918): 451–56.

Stepan, Nancy. "The Interplay between Socio-Economic Factors and Medical Science: Yellow Fever Research, Cuba and the United States." *Social Studies of Science* 8 (November 1978): 397–423.

Sternberg, George. "The Transmission of Yellow Fever by Mosquitoes." *Popular Science Monthly* July 1901 cited in Truby, *Memoir of Walter Reed*, 90.

Sullivan, David J. "Human *Plasmodium Vivax* Mosquito Experimental Transmission." *Journal of Clinical Investigation* 130 (2020): 2800–802. https://jci.me/135794/pdf.

Sydenstricker, Edgar. "Variations in Case Fatality during the Influenza Epidemic of 1918." *Public Health Reports (1896–1970)* 36 (September 9, 1921): 2201–10.

Taubenberger, Jeffery K. "Seeking the 1918 Spanish Influenza Virus." *American Society of Microbiology News* 65 (July 1999).

Taubenberger, Jeffery K. "The Origin and Virulence of the 1918 'Spanish' Influenza Virus." *Proceedings of the American Philosophical Society* 150 (March 2006): 86–112.

Taubenberger, Jeffery K., and David M. Morens. "1918 Influenza: The Mother of All Pandemics." *Emerging Infectious Diseases* 12 (2006): 15–22.

Taubenberger, Jeffery K., et al. "Initial Genetic Characterization of the 1918 'Spanish' Influenza Virus." *Science* 275 (March 21, 1997): 1793–804.

"The Typhoid Outbreak in the United States Military Camps during the Spanish War." *British Medical Journal* 2 (July 1905): 137–40.

"The Anti-Vivisectionists and the Inoculation against Typhoid." *British Medical Journal* 1 (January 1915): 171.

Transylvania Journal of Medicine and the Associate Sciences, November 1830.

Traub, Robert, and Charles Wisseman Jr. "Korean Hemorrhagic Fever." *Journal of Infectious Diseases* 138 (August 1978): 267–72.

U.S. Public Health Service. "Epidemic Influenza: Prevalence in the United States." *Public Health Reports* 33 (November 8, 1918): 1913–21.

Vainio, Jari, and Felicity Cutts. "Yellow Fever. Division of Emerging and Other Communicable Diseases Surveillance and Control." *World Health Organization 1998*. Accessed November 2020. http://www.who.ch/gpv-documents/.

Van Cleave, Harley J. "Returning Service Men a Problem in National Health." *American Scientist* 32 (October 1944): 243–53.

Van Zwanenberg, David. "The Suttons and the Business of Inoculation." *Medical History* 22 (1978): 71–82.

Vaughan, Victor. "Some Remarks on Typhoid Fever among Our Soldiers during the Late War with Spain." *American Journal of the Medical Sciences*. Reprint. Accessed November 10, 2021. https://collections.nlm.nih.gov/bookviewer?PID=nlm:nlmuid-101473324-bk.

Warner, Margaret. "Hunting the Yellow Fever Germ: The Principle and Practice of Etiological Proof in the Late Nineteenth Century." *Bulletin of the History of Medicine* 59 (1985): 361–82.

Wasdin, Eugene, and H. D. Geddings. "The Etiology of Yellow Fever—Abstract of a Report of the Commission of Medical Officers, Marine-Hospital Service, Detailed by Authority of the President to Investigate the Cause of Yellow Fever." *Public Health Reports* 14 (August 18, 1899): 1303–308.

———. "Preliminary Report of Medical Officers Detailed by Direction of the President as a Commission to Investigate in Habana the Cause of Yellow Fever." *Public Health Reports* 13 (November 11, 1898): 1265–76.

Weina, Peter. "From Atabrine in World War II to Mefloquine in Somalia: The Role of Education in Preventive Medicine." *Military Medicine* 163 (September 1998): 635–39.

White, N. J. "Emergence of Artemisinin-Resistant Plasmodium Falciparum in East Africa." *New England Journal of Medicine* 358 (September 23, 2021): 1231–32.

Woodward, J. J. "Typho-Malarial Fever: Is It a Special Type of Fever? Remarks Introductory to the Discussion of the Question, Section of Medicine, International Medical Congress, Philadelphia 1876." Reprint. Accessed November 9, 2021. https://collections.nlm.nih.gov/bookviewer?PID=nlm:nlmuid -9609653-bk.

Worobey, Michael, Guan-Zhu Han, and Andrew Rambaut. "Genesis and Pathogenesis of the 1918 Pandemic H1N1 Influenza Virus." *Proceedings of the National Academy of Sciences of the United States of America* 22 (June 2014): 8107–112.

Worthen, Dennis. "The Natlongstreeional Quinine Pool: When Quinine Went to War." *Pharmacy in History* 38 (1996): 143–47.

PRIMARY SOURCES

Barclay, Harold. *A Doctor in France, 1917–1919.* New York: Privately printed, 1923.

Butterfield, L. H., ed. *Letters of Benjamin Rush.* Philadelphia: American Philosophical Society for Princeton University Press, 1951.

Continental Congress Journals, 1774–1789, Washington, D.C., 1921–26, Vol. II, 92. *Journals of the Continental Congress Home Page: U.S. Congressional Documents* (loc.gov). Accessed July 30, 2021.

Cushing, Harvey. *From a Surgeon's Journal.* Boston: Little, Brown and Company, 1937.

Ireland, M. W. *Report of the Surgeon General, U.S. Army to the Secretary of War, 1919.* Washington, D.C.: Government Printing Office, 1919.

Kean, Jefferson Randolph. "Memoirs." Accessed March 2, 2021. https://medcoeck apwstorprd01.blob.core.usgovcloudapi.net/achh/JeffersonRandolphKean.pdf.

Lada, John, ed. *Medical Statistics in World War II.* Washington, D.C.: Office of the Surgeon General, Department of the Army, 1975.

McGuire, Stuart. *History of U.S. Army Base Hospital No. 45 in the Great War.* Richmond, VA: William Byrd Press, 1924, 252.

"Military Control of Malaria and Insect-Borne Diseases." *Preventive Medicine Manual No. 2 for All Officers.* United States Army Forces, Pacific Ocean Areas, Lt. General Robert C. Richardson Jr., Commanding. June 1945.

National Archives and Records Administration, Founders Documents. https://founders.archives.gov/.

National Archives and Records Administration, Record Group 112: Records of the Office of the Surgeon General.

Owen, William, compiler and ed. *The Medical Department of the United States Army during the Period of the Revolution (1776–1786).* New York: Paul B. Hoeber, 1920.

Philip S. Hench Walter Reed Yellow Fever Collection 1806–1995, Historical Collections, Claude Moore Health Sciences Library, University of Virginia.

Report of the Surgeon General U.S. Army to the Secretary of War: 1919. Washington, D.C.: Government Printing Office, 1919; 38, 42–43, 752.

Richardson, Robert C. "Preventive Medicine Manual No. 2 for All Officers: Military Control of Malaria and Insect-Borne Diseases." *Headquarters United States Army Forces, Pacific Ocean Areas, Office of the Commanding General, APO 958,* June 1945.

Senter, Isaac. *The Journal of Isaac Senter, Physician and Surgeon to the Troops Detached from the American Army Encamped at Cambridge, Mass. On a Secret Expedition against Quebec under the Command of Col. Benedict Arnold in September 1775.* Philadelphia: Historical Society of Pennsylvania, 1846.

U.S. Surgeon General's Office. *Regulations for the Medical Department of the Army.* Washington, D.C.: Government Printing Office, 1861.

Vaughan, Victor C. *Doctor's Memories.* Indianapolis, IN: Bobbs-Merrill Company, 1926.

von Ludendorff, Erich. *Ludendorff's Own Story.* Vol. 2. New York: Harper and Bros., 1919.

"War Department Special Regulation No. 28." *Sanitary Regulations and Control of Communicable Diseases.* Washington, D.C.: Government Printing Office, 1917, 7.

INDEX

ABOUT THE AUTHOR

Jack E. McCallum holds a Bachelor of Science degree from Georgia Institute of Technology, a Master of Arts in history from Texas Christian University, a doctorate in medicine from Emory University, and a doctorate in history from Texas Christian University. He has board certification in both adult and pediatric neurosurgery, has held teaching appointments in medicine and history at several universities, and has been founder and chief executive officer of four successful companies. He has published two books and numerous articles dealing with both medicine and history and taught history at the graduate and undergraduate level for seventeen years.

The **Naval Institute Press** is the book-publishing arm of the U.S. Naval Institute, a private, nonprofit, membership society for sea service professionals and others who share an interest in naval and maritime affairs. Established in 1873 at the U.S. Naval Academy in Annapolis, Maryland, where its offices remain today, the Naval Institute has members worldwide.

Members of the Naval Institute support the education programs of the society and receive the influential monthly magazine *Proceedings* or the colorful bimonthly magazine *Naval History* and discounts on fine nautical prints and on ship and aircraft photos. They also have access to the transcripts of the Institute's Oral History Program and get discounted admission to any of the Institute-sponsored seminars offered around the country.

The Naval Institute's book-publishing program, begun in 1898 with basic guides to naval practices, has broadened its scope to include books of more general interest. Now the Naval Institute Press publishes about seventy titles each year, ranging from how-to books on boating and navigation to battle histories, biographies, ship and aircraft guides, and novels. Institute members receive significant discounts on the Press' more than eight hundred books in print.

Full-time students are eligible for special half-price membership rates. Life memberships are also available.

For more information about Naval Institute Press books that are currently available, visit www.usni.org/press/books. To learn about joining the U.S. Naval Institute, please write to:

Member Services
U.S. Naval Institute
291 Wood Road
Annapolis, MD 21402-5034
Telephone: (800) 233-8764
Fax: (410) 571-1703
Web address: www.usni.org